My Bonnie

My Bonnie

How dementia
stole the love of my life

JOHN
SUCHET

HarperCollins*Publishers*

HarperCollins Publishers
77–85 Fulham Palace Road,
Hammersmith, London W6 8JB

www.harpercollins.co.uk

First published in 2010

1 2 3 4 5 6 7 8 9 10

This is a work of non-fiction. In order to protect privacy,
some names and places have been changed.

John Suchet asserts the moral right to be
identified as the author of this work

A catalogue record of this book is
available from the British Library

HB ISBN 978-0-00-732842-0
PB ISBN 978-0-00-732840-6

Printed and bound in Great Britain by
Clays Ltd, St Ives plc

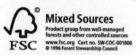

Mum and Dad, with love

Prologue

In the summer of 2004, my wife Bonnie and I were in the departure lounge at Stansted airport, waiting to board the short flight down to our house in the French countryside. Bon said she would just nip to the toilet. 'Fine,' I said, 'but don't be too long. We'll be boarding soon.' She walked off to the ladies, which was not more than 10 metres away.

Five minutes went by, 10, then 15. I was beginning to get seriously concerned. Mild worry turned into panic. I looked long and hard at the entrance to the ladies. I decided I would ask the next woman who emerged to go back in and call Bonnie's name. I imagined the worst, as you do. A heart attack, a stroke, and … No, it didn't bear thinking about.

A woman came out. It wasn't Bonnie. I began to move towards her, when suddenly I heard, clear as a bell and reverberating from wall to wall, *'Would Mr Suchet, Mr John Suchet, please come to the information desk?'*

I saw a hundred, no a thousand – make that a million – faces turn towards me. (It was probably about six, but it felt like a million.) I hurried to the desk, expecting to find police, paramedics, who knew what else? My breathing was quick and shallow and I felt nausea in my stomach.

Suddenly there she was. Bonnie. Standing at the information desk, looking totally fine. The panic turned in an instant into relief – and a dose of anger. What on earth was she thinking of? Why in heaven's name had she come to the information desk, when I was waiting just a few yards away?

But then she saw me, and her face lit up with a beatific smile, which spelled relief from ear to ear. 'There you are! Thank goodness! I thought I had lost you!' she said.

I took her by the arm and led her, perhaps a touch too firmly, back to the gate, trying at the same time to work out how she had managed to get past without me seeing her. Then I remembered there were two exits, one on the other side.

'What was all that about? Why did you have me paged? I was waiting for you right here.' There was anger in my voice, and I couldn't disguise it. I looked at her, and she was frowning, but it was not a frown of annoyance – it was a frown of non-comprehension. 'I don't understand,' she said. That struck me as odd. It's not what you would expect her to say. *'Don't be angry ... I made a mistake, that's all. Let it go, please.'* Anything like that would be the normal response. But *'I don't understand'* – that's not what you'd expect.

I said nothing more. We boarded the plane. I sat back in the seat and thought the whole incident through. I couldn't make sense of it. All I knew, deep down, was that it shouldn't have happened.

We got to France and I quickly forgot about it. I shouldn't have. It was the beginning.

Chapter 1

27th April 1983

Bonnie and I are going to be together at last. I was up at dawn, tidying the bedsit of which I am so irrationally proud. We both had large houses in the English countryside, but I think I love this bedsit more than anywhere I have ever lived. Before breakfast I polished the kitchen and bathroom floors on my knees, then vacuumed the rugs in the main room. After breakfast I went out to the florist and bought some flowers. I didn't know what to get. The girl said, May I ask what they are for? I grinned from ear to ear. To welcome someone very special, er, a woman. She smiled knowingly and selected something. I can't remember what she chose. As I left the shop, clutching the bouquet awkwardly, I realised I had nothing to put it in. I went back in. She laughed. I bought a small green vase, pinched at the middle, with slanted ripples in the glass. It is on the sideboard and I am looking at it now as I write this, 26 years later.

I drive to Baltimore Washington International airport in the office Volvo, cursing the traffic that has made me a little late. I park and run towards the arrivals terminal, praying she has not come through. I don't see her at first, then I realise it is her. A slim figure standing outside the doors. She is wearing a long summer skirt and coloured short-sleeved top. She has her hand on the extended handle of a suitcase. On top of the suitcase is an open wicker bag. Then I realise why I hadn't at first recognised her. On her head she is wearing a straw hat. Round it are large multi-coloured paper flowers. The hat has cast her face into shadow.

I stop and look at her. She seems so frail. She has lost weight. Those wonderful high cheekbones give her face a fragile beauty. My breath quickens and my heart beats more strongly. My Bonnie is here. She has come to live with me. Her smile when she sees me is nervous, but it lights up her face.

In the car we are silent. I turn to her a couple of times. Each time she returns my smile, but I can sense the anxiety. Why are you anxious? I ask, cursing myself for the stupid question. I'm just a bit nervous, she says. I try to comfort her with a smile.

We walk along the corridor, and I open the door to my bedsit. The first real test. What will she say? Will she like it? Will she recoil in horror at the smallness of it? But I'm not really worried. She throws her arms out, does a twirl, and says it's lovely.

I fold her up in my arms, breathe her in, stroke her skin. I look into her eyes as her eyelids slowly close and she turns her face up to mine.

In the evening, as she prepares a simple dinner, I open a bottle of sparkling wine and we toast the future. I spread a green cloth over a small table, both given to me by my camera crew. She takes two candleholders and two slim white candles out of the wicker bag, places them on the table and lights them.

With slight trepidation (not all women like being photographed at a moment's notice), I ask her if she would mind if I took a photograph. I never want to forget this moment, I say. Of course not, she says, giving the ends of her hair a little flick. I set up my old mechanical Nikon on some boxes and books, activate the self-timer, and run back to the table. One day, I say to her, I will write our story, and this photo will be on the cover. And now it is.

Her name is Bonnie, and no, it is not short for anything. Her father named her after Rhett and Scarlett's young daughter in *Gone With The Wind*. (She came to a sticky end, but we'll let that go.) He named his only daughter Bonnie because he liked the name, simple as that. Bonnie herself has not always been so fond of it. When she worked in London for an international charitable foundation, she complained to me that most people called her Bunny. Pointing out her name was actually Bonnie didn't improve things much; the damage was done, and she believed they didn't take her seriously. I have always adored the name. It is understated, friendly and instantly likeable.

She was born in New Jersey in 1941, and if you want a comparison for her in her younger years, think Grace Kelly in *High Society*, the archetypal elegant and cool American East Coast blonde. For a later comparison, the actress Lee Remick will do. In the years when I pined hopelessly for her and she relished my company only in my fertile imagination, I contented myself by putting her alongside Grace and Lee, my trio of American blondes, all utterly lovely and utterly unattainable. Don't be too hard on me; a man is allowed his fantasy.

So the fact that she is beautiful is incontrovertible. It is simply a fact. A cursory glance at some of the photographs in this book will be enough to convince any doubter, but if you demand further proof, then brace yourself for this: by the time she was 20 years of age Bonnie was four times beauty queen. Not once, twice, or even three times, but *four* times. At each school she attended she was voted beauty queen and, most prestigious of all, at Cornell University she was crowned Homecoming Queen.

In case you should form the wrong opinion, I would like to stress that in not a single case did she put herself forward for these contests. In the early years it was a combination of school and parents, and at Cornell it was the students themselves who chose her. Not much upsets my Bonnie, but in years gone by if ever I wanted to make her just that tiny little bit fractious, I would remind her she was four times beauty queen.

'No, stop that,' she would say, 'you're embarrassing me.' I would gently josh her, force that radiant smile to emerge, then hug her till it hurt.

In her final year at Cornell, she and a small group of female friends came to Europe to explore the Old World. The young men of Italy, Spain, France, thought all their Christmases had come at once – I know so because she told me that one day one of the other women said to her, 'If you get another one tonight, could you pass him on to me'. But Bonnie left them to nurse damaged hearts – except in England, where one persistent suitor was ultimately to be rewarded. She went back to Cornell, but after graduation Bonnie returned to London and married her Englishman.

She later told me that from the day she set foot in England she felt as if she was returning home. Everything about the old country appealed to her, and she knew immediately she would make it her home. As I write this, she has lived in the UK for more than 40 years.

* * * *

You don't need to know much about me, so I will keep it brief. I was born in central London in 1944, the eldest son of a much-respected gynaecologist and obstetrician. Today I live with Bonnie in the same block of flats in which I spent the first 10 years of my life (two doors away on the same floor).

My school career was remarkable for its ordinariness. I made a lot of noise and achieved very little. At prep school I was caned relentlessly, along with my brother David, by a sadistic headmaster. At public school I was punished by a narrow-minded music director for playing jazz on school premises. I was relatively good at modern languages – French, German, Russian – and taught myself to play trombone to quite a high standard (which led to the offending jazz session). I managed to fail or achieve only mediocre passes in all exams, even in my stronger subjects, but a fortunate phone call at the right moment to the right faculty earned me a place at university. It was in Dundee, which shocked my parents, and we had to look at Dad's AA road map of the UK to find out where it was. Four years later I was a Master of Arts (with Honours) but, more importantly, I had secured a position as graduate trainee with Reuters news agency in Fleet Street, London.

I will not bore on about exactly how I achieved that, other than to say that it was a combination of a certain ease in writing a news story, combined with a shameless exaggeration of my linguistic skills, which at interview were never put to the test. Just recently, around 40 years on, I was host at a social event in the City of London, at which the two former Reuters executives (long since retired) who had interviewed me were present. In my speech I finally confessed to them that had they tested my claims as a linguist, I would have been on the next train north. There was much laughter, and a few good-natured boos.

The start to my Reuters career was stellar. Eight months after joining – a year since my graduation – I was on the streets of Paris, covering the student riots of 1968, which ultimately led to the downfall of President de Gaulle. But, true to form, I then proceeded to make a mess of things by turning down the opportunity to become bureau chief in Congo Brazzaville. (It was a startling promotion, but my then wife insisted we needed to stay in the UK to look for a house and take out a mortgage. So I turned down Brazzaville, knowing I was making the first major mistake of my fledgling journalistic career.) I resigned, failed to find another job, then a fortunate phone call to the right person at the right time landed me a lowly job in BBC television news, writing the football results and weather forecasts. I managed to do even that quite badly, and after a year-and-a-half left for ITN, telling the BBC I would be back in a year. I stayed at ITN for the rest of my career. In 2008 the Royal Television Society presented me with a Lifetime Achievement Award, its highest accolade. I don't know why – I'm convinced they got the wrong person – and when I look at the very smart gold and engraved glass award sitting on my grandparents' glass-fronted cabinet, I regularly say to Bonnie that when they realise their mistake it'll be too late, they're not getting it back.

Back at the beginning of 1970, with my career in tatters, my first wife Moya and I moved into a Victorian cottage at the end of a cul-de-sac in leafy Henley-on-Thames and I took on a crippling mortgage. The house was cold and damp and parts of it were at risk of falling down. It needed a lot of work, and I had never held a drill in my life. A small slope went up into woods opposite our house. Three new houses had been built on it, red brick, boxlike, unattractive. In the summer of 1970, Bonnie and her husband moved into the house at the top of the slope.

I am writing this at the large oak dining table in the old farmhouse Bonnie and I bought 20 years ago in Gascony in south-west France. Bonnie is walking slowly around the house. It's what she does now. She can't settle. She stands at the kitchen door, squinting at the brightness outside. She walks the length of the kitchen, then into the sitting room, which we call the *séjour*, where I am writing. Hello darling, I say, I am writing about you. Good, she says, without questioning me any further. On the table is a large brown envelope with my name on it. Inside are sample chapters of a forth-coming book in which carers tell their stories of caring for a loved one with dementia. The author has asked me to write a short paragraph endorsing the book. Bonnie picks up the envelope, but I am not worried she will open it or even ask what is in it. Have you seen this, she asks?

Yes, I say, affecting a slight weariness in my voice. It's from a charity I am doing some work for. They want me to read it and give my comments. Lot of stuff to get through. She smiles and puts it down, and walks back to the kitchen, where she stands at the door and squints her eyes again at the brightness outside.

I haven't lied to her, I have told her something which is very close to the truth and which I know she will be comfortable with. I am getting better at entering her world and only saying things I know she will comprehend. I mustn't try to take her outside her world. The tragedy is that that world is slowly shrinking, so something she may grasp today may elude her tomorrow. I have to be on the lookout for that.

I said she doesn't settle. It is strange, and at first – for some time, in fact – I found it irritating and rather wearying. Why don't you sit down, love? Sit in an armchair and relax. All right, she would say, and continue her gentle pacing. *Do not try to take her outside her world.* So now I say nothing. She is content. But I do have the power to alter things. If I close the computer now, get up, say I have finished writing, and go and sit in an armchair, she will come and sit in an armchair with me.

She has been patiently pacing for the last couple of hours while I have been filling you in on my unillustrious past, so the time has come to stop and give some time to her. So if you'll excuse me …

My first wife Moya and I had a volatile, combustive relationship. Although from totally different backgrounds, our temperaments were rather similar. We were both highly strung, emotional, quick to judgment, with a temper. She came from a Scottish family and was proud of her Celtic blood. I came from, er, lots of different places. Yet we were both, to simplify, 'artists' rather than 'scientists'. We liked books, theatre, films, music. Only problem was we liked totally different books, theatre, films, music to each other. There would be fierce argument about the merits or de-merits of a particular work of art, with measures of intolerance and ridicule thrown in. There was rarely a meeting of minds.

I was 19 when we met and 24 when we married. Ridiculously young, really, but I was the product of a 'boys only' education. At prep school the most popular boys were the ones who had a sister who just might come to visit, which would mean a rare sighting of a sublime creature with long hair wearing a skirt and maybe – god, the thrill of expectation

— a touch of lipstick. At public school we were expressly forbidden from talking to girls who lived in the town. A boy who had the temerity not only to do that but to date her as well, was expelled between making the date and keeping it. How then to get to know these wonderful creatures? How to approach them, what on earth to say to them? For me even at 18, girls were mysterious and desirable creatures from another planet. I had no idea how to talk to one, let alone how to embark on anything more daring. And so practically the first girl who (finally) allowed me to kiss her became my wife.

My parents could see that, in marrying Moya, I was about to make the mistake of my life. Both tried hard to talk sense into me, to make me change my mind. Does a very young man who has secured an Honours degree in Political Science and Philosophy, who has landed the job of a lifetime at the first attempt, listen to his parents? Some may, but this one did not.

Problem was, Moya knew full well the lengths my parents had gone to in their attempts to stop me marrying her, and so once we were married she insisted I was to have nothing more to do with them. *Nothing.* I wasn't to see them, or try to make contact with them in any way. I had a new life now, with her. Even I could see that was a bit extreme, but I let it go. Emotions were running high. I thought in time they would settle on both sides, and life would get back to normal. But it didn't. She really meant it. I soon learned that even to mention my parents was to invite trouble. Still I did nothing to correct the situation. The birth of our first son, Damian, did little to calm things down. I threw myself into my work, and when we moved out to Henley it put physical distance between me and my 'old' family. Always at the back of my mind was the belief that one day matters would correct themselves, but in the meantime it simply became easier to carry on doing nothing. It made for an easier life.

Two more sons, Kieran and Rory, arrived, but I wasn't allowed to tell their grandparents, never mind take them for a visit. How much longer would this new way of life last? I clung to the belief that it might end at any moment. My worst nightmare was that one of my parents would die before it was rectified. I felt guilty that I was allowing it to happen, but couldn't think how to resolve it without damaging my increasingly strained marriage.

Meanwhile, my attention had been caught by the young blonde woman who lived in the house at the top of the slope. I had found out her name was Bonnie. She was stunningly beautiful and around her shone an aura of calm. Even before I had exchanged anything more than social pleasantries with her, I knew profoundly, totally, with not a shred of doubt or hesitation, that this would be my ideal woman. Sadly, a woman who could never belong to me. Too bad. I wouldn't be the first man to find himself in such a position. At the very least, I thought, I would enjoy getting to know her, and derive pleasure from that.

✳ ✳ ✳ ✳

Dreams are cruel and memories hurt. Just before waking this morning, I had the most intense dream about Bonnie. The old days were back. You can imagine. I awoke to feel her getting out of bed and knew I would have to lead her to the bathroom. Black dog depression on my shoulders. I got her dressed, and saw hanging up one of her favourite tops, colourful, beautiful, elegant. Boy, she used to turn heads when she wore that. It has been untouched for years. There is no point in reminding her of it – she would just smile and say yes. I touched it, as I used to, and stroked the buttons I was once so expert at loosening.

At breakfast she stood and walked to the kitchen door. She chuckled and said in a mock Cockney accent, 'Is that your car?' 'Sorry?' I asked. She repeated it, adding, 'You know, that's what those people say, those people, you know the ones, they just came in.' I laughed and agreed. In fact, it is an annoying ad running on UK television at the moment, and she has memorised the catchphrase.

Good start to the day, triple whammy depression. I snap myself out of it, repeating the mantra – no self-pity, John, no self-pity. But it is so difficult. Here she is again now, just walking in and out of the *séjour*, while I tap-tap away, conjuring her up in my mind as she was in those long-gone, distant days, when I responded to her every word, every casually administered gesture. In my mind there is one person, in front of my eyes another, different person. It is impossible to stop the tears.

* * * *

Bonnie and I met socially over the years, as neighbours do. When we were together my senses were heightened, my brain was more alert, my wit quicker, my conversation more sparkling (at least I thought so). She would respond with a serene and gentle smile, and softly spoken words. I thrilled at her accent, the anglicised American tones, the long 'a's and audible 'r's. Nothing dramatic or obvious. With Bonnie, everything was soft, gentle, subtle. Later, I would relive every word she had said to me. Was there a message, a sign? Was she trying to tell me something secret and important? Of course not, you fool.

At a dinner party at her house some time in the early to mid seventies, I saw a framed photograph of her with three smiling young men. I asked who they were. 'My brothers,' she replied. At the back of the group, the tallest had a strikingly handsome face, prematurely greying hair and neat beard. 'You look so like him,' I said. Her face lit up. 'That's Bob, the eldest. I'm next.' 'Nice looking,' I said, 'you all are.' (Bold, I remember thinking, maybe too bold.) To my delight she began to talk about her family. She told me that her father was an executive with US Steel, which had meant moving the family across the US. She told me she had been born in Jersey City, but had lived in Maryland, Alabama, California. 'In fact, it's quite sad about Bob,' she continued. 'He really loved it in California. We lived in Whittier, just outside Los Angeles –' 'Nixon,' I interjected, 'he came from there.' (Shut up, you fool, let her speak.) She nodded. 'He was doing so well in school, he was academically bright, he was captain of the football team, he had a lovely girlfriend. But then US Steel wanted Dad to come back east. It was a huge wrench for Bob. He kind of gave up, he stopped trying. But he's fine now. He's got a lovely wife. In fact, one day you must meet my brothers. They're bound to come over sooner or later.'

I can't remember much more of what she said. I just wanted her to go on speaking and never stop.

✳ ✳ ✳ ✳

In December 2008 there was a family wedding in Haddonfield, New Jersey. Bonnie's nephew – son of her youngest brother – was getting married. I was worried about making the journey because of Bon's health. Also it would mean staying in a hotel, with all the confusion that would bring. But it was vitally important we attend. Bon's eldest brother Bob was terminally ill with oesophageal cancer. He had undergone several bouts of chemotherapy, but his lungs were filling up, requiring regular draining. The doctors had sent him home and warned the family he didn't have long to live.

We went, and Bonnie coped better than I expected. There were a couple of middle-of-the-night excursions into the hotel corridor, but nothing I couldn't handle. What really surprised me, though, was how Bon reacted to Bob's illness. He was, frankly, in an appalling state. Skin and bone, protruding spine, sunken face, staringly bright eyes. I hugged him, and he let out a shout – I had pushed the permanently inserted catheter against his ribs. But Bon didn't seem overly distressed. In one extraordinarily poignant moment, I saw her holding his hand and heard her telling him he must get better.

Thank goodness we made the journey. Bob died two months later. I haven't told Bon. Why make her sad? She doesn't need to know.

✳ ✳ ✳ ✳

Things definitely changed some time around 1978. There was a big dinner party, about a dozen of us, all local couples, and we held it in a fancy restaurant, the French Horn in Sonning. I found myself sitting next to Bonnie, with both our spouses a fair distance away on the other side of the table. She had swept her blonde hair back from her face and held it in place with two cream combs. I don't think I had ever seen anything more lovely. It set off her face in all its beauty, her peach skin and sparkling eyes vibrant and alive. I was in heaven. We chatted together right through the meal. God knows who was on my left or her right, but they might as well not have existed. It was the longest I had ever spoken to her for, and I wasn't going to waste a second of it.

I could say my wit was at its sparkling best, and you would groan and roll your eyes, but really it was. Late on in the meal, she was asking me about my job. I told her I was an ITN reporter and mentioned one or two stories I had covered, and she said she had seen me on *News at Ten*. I was flattered. I wanted to ask her what she thought, but decided not to put her on the spot.

Then she said, and I remember it perfectly more than 30 years later, 'Aren't journalists supposed to be rottweilers?' I laughed and replied, 'Well, not me, I'm just a poodle.' She burst into uncontrollable laughter. She threw her head back, her hair cascaded round her face, dancing below the combs. Then her head came forward, shimmering tears of laughter in her eyes. She put her hand on my arm to steady herself, but still her laughter shook her body, a sound more beautiful and joyous than any I had heard. I glanced quickly around the table – all heads had turned. Still she laughed, looking me in the eye now. Very slowly her laughter began to subside, but her cheeks were flushed, her eyes still fiery bright. She took a swallow of water. 'You are funny,' she said, and looked at me in a way I cannot describe. There was something new about it, something intimate.

I will wind the clock forward 10 or 12 years. We were by now married, and having dinner with a business colleague of Bonnie's and his wife.

Bonnie looked stunning in a dark skirt and colourful shaped blouse that showed her off to perfection. Her lovely hair was again pulled back and held in place by those two cream combs. 'How did you two meet?' the man's wife asked. Bon shot me a look. She always felt slightly uncomfortable if I said we had been neighbours, and had asked me in the past to say something to the effect that we were introduced by friends, something neutral which should not lead to more questioning.

I said, 'We were in a crowded room, our eyes met, I said Ugh, she said Ugh, and that was that – we are not very good with words.' Bon did that laugh again. It was an exact repeat of the French Horn. She threw her head back and laughed until her ribs hurt. I laughed with her. The man and his wife looked at each other and joined in the laughter, but not very fully. I caught a look she gave him, which sort of said, 'Why can't you make me laugh like that?'

On the way home, Bon said she loved what I had said, she would never forget that it all began when we said Ugh to each other, and we laughed together all over again. Those combs are in a drawer of her dressing-table in our flat to this day. Just a few months ago, I saw her walking around the flat with them in her hand. She didn't put them in her hair, just carried them around, occasionally putting them in her cardigan pocket, then taking them out again. I didn't say anything. If I had said, Do you remember how I used to love you wearing those, she would just have said yes. But she wouldn't remember really, and it might cause her a little pain deep down because she would know she doesn't really remember. Later she put them back in the drawer and hasn't taken them out since.

* * * *

'I am writing about you, my Bonnie.'

'Oh are you? That's nice,' and she walks away.

* * * *

There was a subtle change one summer's evening in, I think, 1979. Bonnie and her husband invited my wife and me up to their house for dinner. Don't think me vain, but I can remember exactly what I was wearing that night, and for good reason. I had on a dark blue blazer, open neck blue shirt and new pale blue slacks. We arrived a little early (probably my fault), the back door was open, and Bonnie called down to us to make ourselves at home in the sitting room, that she and her husband would be down in a minute.

There was a news journal on the coffee table. I picked it up and flicked through it. Aware that she would walk through the door at any moment, I affected insouciance, standing in relaxed manner, weight on one leg, the other informally outstretched, not taking in a single word on the printed page in front of me, hoping I was striking an irresistibly alluring image. The minutes passed. Finally I heard the light footsteps approaching, I adjusted my pose slightly – back that little bit straighter, biceps slightly flexed, one eyebrow subtly raised, nostrils marginally flared, a look of utterly false concentration on my face as I affected to be studying a learned article about something happening somewhere in the world. She walked in. I raised my head slowly and at an angle, a Cary Grant smile playing on one corner of my mouth, hoping it would strike the perfect combination of intelligence and pleasurably interrupted concentration.

'Ooh look,' she cooed, 'John all dishy in blue.'

I chuckled in a manly way and flicked my head so a lock of hair fell springily onto my forehead. Rather that's what I wished I had done. In fact I half-dropped the journal, slightly lost my balance on the supporting leg, caught my breath so I nearly choked, and all round made a pretty damn fool of myself.

But she said it, she really did say it. I remember the words exactly, and can even hear her tone of voice – mild, pleasurable and seductive – 30 years on. After that, I spent the evening in a sort of daze. I can't remember anything of how the dinner went, what we talked about, except that I recall running those few words through my head again and again and again. Why did she say it? What did it mean? Was she trying to say something more? Was it, in fact, a subtle way of saying something else?

I knew I was fooling myself. The answers to all these stupid questions were pretty obvious. She said it on the spur of the moment, without pausing for thought. But that in itself was amazing enough: it meant she really thought it. If she hadn't thought it, she wouldn't have said it. I reasoned that much, so I probably spent the rest of the evening with a foolish and rather smug grin on my face.

There was more to come. When it came time to say goodnight, Bonnie and her husband escorted us out of the front door. It was a warm rather sultry evening. It was customary to administer a French-style peck on both cheeks. She and I had done it a dozen times at various social functions. I moved towards Bonnie, she moved towards me, and as I leaned forward she didn't turn her head, so I kissed her on the lips. Just fleetingly, no more than a split second. But all the clichés happened. A shaft of heat shot through my body, a mini-explosion went off in my head, my mouth hung half open, a smile spread from ear to ear. I let her go, I couldn't repeat it, but as she drew back her eyes didn't leave mine.

Now I really did have a question to ask myself. Was that deliberate? I lay in bed that night asking the question, I awoke the next morning still asking the question, and continued to ask it for the next several months, during which I did not see her. It had to be, didn't it? Would a woman accidentally do that? Surely not.

You will not be surprised to learn that some years later, when we were at last together, I asked her the question. I didn't expect her even to remember the occasion, let alone what happened, so I began at the beginning, as it were, by reminding her we had arrived a little early and I was standing reading the news journal. 'And I said John all dishy in blue,' she interrupted. 'Yes, and when we left at the end of the evening ...', 'I kissed you on the lips,' she said.

* * * *

15

My parents were totally out of the picture. Not totally out of my mind, but Moya didn't know that. I had successfully sublimated the guilt, so that as far as she was concerned my life revolved exclusively round my 'new' family.

There were jolts. I was crossing a footbridge at South Kensington tube station one day, and there was a huge poster that said, 'Honour thy Father and Mother'. I swallowed hard and cursed the interfering group of religious bigots that had put it up. I would dream of Mum and Dad, and wake with a leaden feeling of guilt in my head. Then, at a social gathering one Christmas at the home of a mutual friend who lived in the same road, Bonnie and I were engaged in polite conversation. I think we were talking about Watergate, President Ford's outrageous pardon of his predecessor, something like that anyway, when – clearly intending no more than a continuation of chat – unwittingly Bonnie rocked me to the foundations. She asked me about my family, my parents. Nothing abnormal about that, except to someone in my situation. I tried to think quickly of something appropriate to say, something that would sound fine and lead to no further questioning. But what came out was 'I, er, I don't see my parents.' I prayed she would simply move the conversation on, but she was appalled. She repeated what I had said, pausing between each word.

'But that's awful,' she said, 'really awful. Oh, I am so sad for you.'

I felt tears well up in me. Unwittingly she had broken through the defensive wall I had so carefully constructed around me. I knew it was wrong, she knew it was wrong, but I didn't know what to do about it. This particular boat most certainly did not need rocking. It would sink, and I would sink with it.

* * * *

October 1980. Bonnie's husband, an economist, was away on a business trip. Moya and I invited her down to ours for the evening so she wouldn't be on her own. I offered Bonnie a pre-dinner drink and replenished it despite her protestations. She and her husband had recently returned from a trip to Sri Lanka. Bon said she had found the atmosphere there almost erotic. The sultry heat, she said, and the people walking so languidly, their hips swaying and their loose clothing swaying too, men and women alike.

I don't know about bloody Sri Lanka, but hearing Bonnie talk like that was pretty damn erotic for me. My imagination soared and the thought of Bonnie becoming aroused, combined most certainly with a strong scotch and soda, brought a crimson heat to my face which I made no attempt to conceal. I probably spent the rest of the evening grinning like the proverbial Cheshire cat. After all, I was in close proximity to a calm, softly spoken, gentle woman who had begun to fill my waking thoughts, and most of my nightly ones as well.

Some time around the middle of the evening, the heavens opened and the rain came bucketing down. It pounded on the roof and we could hear it splashing off the pavement outside. Throughout the evening, I made sure Bon's wine glass was never empty, although I noticed she wised up to this quickly and never had more than a sip or two before I wielded the bottle again. Finally she said she ought to get back home and relieve the babysitter, who was looking after her two children. My wife nodded. Then she said, and these were her exact words, 'John, you're not going to let Bonnie walk home alone, are you, in this pouring rain? You must go with her.'

I swallowed hard. 'Of course,' I said, as a thousand butterflies suddenly took flight in my stomach. I remember the feeling. If this had been a movie, the camera would have caught the smug smile of satisfaction as I realised this was the moment I had waited for for so long. In fact, the feeling that filled me was closer to panic. What should I do? How should I behave? What if, in the next few minutes, it became transparently clear to me that Bonnie had no more feeling for me than any other bloke she had come into contact with? The illusion, the fictional edifice I had built, would be fatally breached and come tumbling down.

Oh Lordy, oh God, oh Hell, I thought as I took the umbrella my wife handed to me. We stepped outside, the two of us, making small exclamatory noises as the rain hit us. Bonnie took a hurried couple of steps to the gate before I could get the umbrella up. Rejection. Obvious. Fool. I hurried after her and onto the pavement. She waited for me to catch up. Ha! Good sign. Or not. The street lamp lit up her face as she half turned, the rain soaking her and drops rolling down her cheeks. She was smiling a wide smile.

'Here,' I said, 'come under the umbrella.' I raised it over her head and in a move that seemed as natural as breathing, I put my arm round her. She allowed me to draw her body closer to me. We walked that way up the slope to her house, in step with each other and laughing like teenagers. We reached the back door of her house. A dim light came from inside, but apart from that we were in darkness. The overhanging roof gave us slight shelter from the rain, but not much.

I put down the umbrella and reached out to her. Her arms reached out to me. We took a step towards each other and our lips locked in a moment of the most intense passion I had ever felt. We kissed as though our lives depended on it. I parted her lips with my tongue, she responded and she pressed herself fully against me. I tasted her, inhaled her scent. I stroked her body with my hands, feeling up and down her back, the indent of her waist, then, gently, the contours of her front. She made small gasping sounds, seeming to crave me as much as I craved her. I felt her hands on my back, my neck, my head.

I don't know how long that immortal first kiss lasted. Minutes, certainly. In the movie I would have told her how I loved her, how I had longed for her, how I had waited for this moment. She would have sighed ecstatically, returned my ardent words, probably to the strains of

Rachmaninov. In fact, we said nothing. Our eyes held each other for a few moments. I picked up the umbrella and walked back down the slope.

* * * *

I have thought about this moment a million times in the more than 30 years since it happened. Bonnie and I have talked about it, laughed over it. It has always led to a repeat performance. Today, as I write about it for the first time, it only brings tears to my eyes.

Bonnie is pacing round the house and I want to tell her what I am remembering, but I don't. Why talk of something that will mean nothing to her now, and might make her regret that she can't remember it?

But can I really be sure it will mean nothing to her? What if I am wrong, and she does remember it? If she does, it will bring her a lot of pleasure. I decide to test it in as gentle a way as I can.

I go out onto the terrace, and of course Bon follows me out there. We stroll around for a few moments, then I lean against the table and say, 'Come here, darling, come here a moment.' 'Why?' 'I want to ask you something.'

She walks towards me and stands facing me.

'Do you remember our first kiss?'

'Of course I do.'

'When was it?'

'Er … I don't know.'

'Take a guess.'

'Five years ago?'

'Yeah!' I say, raising my arms in triumph. She smiles with satisfaction.

Chapter 2

So what did it all mean? It seemed impossible that she might actually be interested in me. Let's look at the facts. She – a White Anglo-Saxon Protestant born and educated in America. *Moi* – a rather dark-skinned (olive, I think, is the polite word) Londoner of slightly indeterminate European origin, from around half a dozen Central and Eastern European countries, at least if you go back a couple of generations or so, with a bit of English thrown in, and a totally British upbringing. We had nothing in common, absolutely nothing. Besides, she was married with two sons, to a decent man who, as far as I knew, was a caring father and husband, with a prestigious job that allowed him to provide them with a comfortable life. In short, Bonnie and I were physically, mentally, in every which way possible, polar opposites. What could possibly happen between us, ever?

Soon after we were finally together, I put these facts to her, in a desperate attempt to try to understand her folly. 'Look,' I said, 'I am utterly different to you, in origin, in looks, probably in everything.' 'So?' she countered. I wasn't going to be put off. 'All right, I'm not a blonde, blue-eyed Adonis, you can't argue against that.' 'No, I can't,' she said. 'But I don't want a blonde blue-eyed Adonis.' 'Right,' I replied, gearing myself up for what I knew would be the knockout punch, 'I am not six-foot two. OK? However you look at it, I am not bloody six-foot two. Not even on a good day.' 'So?' she said, moving towards me. 'Look,' and she nestled her head neatly between my upper chest and my neck. 'We are a perfect fit.'

＊ ＊ ＊ ＊

'Darling, would you like some more tomatoes?'

'I like tomatoes, all right? I like them. But I can't eat them now while I'm having this lunch.'

'Fine, darling.'

* * * *

I couldn't have known just how perfect the fit would be, in everything, absolutely everything, physical, mental and emotional. But before I relate how we began to discover that, I need to fill you in on the developments in my glittering career. For once, just once, it really was beginning to glitter.

I had joined ITN in the summer of 1972 in the same lowly capacity as at the BBC, only this time I managed to get the weather forecast and football results mostly right. I was soon promoted from junior scriptwriter to chief sub-editor, but my heart lay in reporting. More than anything else I wanted to be a reporter, to travel the world reporting for *News at Ten*, to be a 'fireman', to use the journalistic term – to go into work in the morning not knowing where in the world I would be that evening. After three years ITN announced it had a vacancy for a reporter, and would accept external as well as internal applications. I was pretty sure I stood no chance, but I also knew if I didn't put in for it, I could kiss my ambitions goodbye. I applied. I did a camera test. I read yesterday's news bulletin. I got the job.

When I left ITN 30 or so years later, my colleagues made a leaving video for me. They unearthed that camera test. A very young me, long hair halfway down to my shoulders, sideburns almost down to my chin, tinted glasses that went automatically darker under the studio lights, wide lapels. Very 1970s, very self-conscious, very gauche. No wonder it was years before Bonnie deigned to afford me a second glance.

The reporting went well, because I loved doing it. Do a job you love, and it's hard to mess it up. 'Suchet delivers,' said the senior foreign desk editor. I did indeed travel the world. I covered the Iran revolution, the Soviet invasion of Afghanistan. I was sent on an impossible mission to the teeming city of Algiers to find an Arab terrorist wanted for masterminding the Munich Olympics massacre: I found him and got an exclusive interview. One boring Sunday afternoon I sat at the reporters' desk, twiddling my thumbs; three hours later I was on a chartered executive jet, flying to Spain to cover a hostage crisis. I attended the last Rhodesian Independence Ball before the country became Zimbabwe. In the late 1970s I came to know Belfast and Derry nearly as well as I knew London. My passport and contact lens solution were always in my briefcase.

Then the plum came up, the most important and prestigious position open to an ITN reporter: US correspondent, based in Washington; ITN's only overseas posting. Back in 1973, as a junior scriptwriter, I had been sent to Washington to act as runner for the then US correspondent, as President Nixon became engulfed in the Watergate scandal. It was my first trip to the United States, and from the day I entered the ITN office, I coveted the job of US correspondent. It was not only an unrealistic ambition, it was an impossible one. No mere scriptwriter had ever become a reporter at ITN, let alone US correspondent. Well, I had achieved the first part of that impossible dream, and now the ultimate prize was open.

I applied for it, and got it. The then editor of ITN, David Nicholas, wrote me a letter telling me the job was mine, and expressing his assurance that I would bring the same distinction to it that I had shown as a general news reporter.

Of course I would. I had wanted this job for the best part of a decade. I had achieved the impossible. Now I would really show what I was capable of. Well, I certainly did that. I proceeded to make such a hash of it that it almost brought my career to a total halt. Doesn't that have a rather familiar ring to it?

* * * *

Yes, yours truly, ace reporter and superstar John Suchet, was about to prove, once again, how when offered his dream on a plate, he repaid his employers' faith in him by messing it up. Big time. I had brought my career at Reuters to a halt with the decision to resign rather than take the job as bureau chief in Brazzaville. It was at Moya's urging, but ultimately it was my decision. After that I almost got myself sacked by the BBC because my work was sloppy and careless, my attitude arrogant. But I came to my senses in time and just as the BBC was applauding my new-found commitment, I cut my losses and moved to ITN. Two damned close-run things had concentrated my mind, and when I began my career at ITN I was utterly determined not to fail. A third disaster would surely mean curtains for this fledgling journalistic career.

I developed a sort of mantra. In my early years at ITN, I would walk through tube stations on my way to work repeating in my head *At ITN I have so far, at ITN I have so far, at ITN I have so far* … It was a way of saying to myself that although things were going well *so far*, I shouldn't be arrogant because it could all go wrong tomorrow. I remember consciously deciding not to say anything as foolish as *At ITN I will*, or *At ITN I have* … That would be tempting fate.

Now, nine years or so into my career at ITN, it really did look as though *I had so far*. Ah yes, so much success, from junior writer to senior writer, to reporter, to correspondent. I truly didn't stop to give those insignificant little words *so far* another thought. But things were soon to become very bad indeed.

In the early months of 1981, I prepared myself and my family for the move to the US, scheduled for July. My three boys were aged 10, seven and five. Moya and I needed to sort out schooling, rent our house out, arrange shipment, and so on. It would be a mammoth task. But hey, in 1979 I had earned plaudits for my coverage of the Iran Revolution (had I not flown from Paris to Tehran with Ayatollah Khomeini?), then I had returned to a greatly changed Tehran to report on the American hostage crisis, as the new Islamic Republic of Iran under the Ayatollah flexed its muscle. At the beginning of 1980, it was off to Afghanistan to cover the Soviet invasion. I went into Afghanistan no fewer than five times, the last three with the Mujahedin, dressed as one of them. Once, my camera crew and I found ourselves in front of what we thought was a Soviet firing squad, up against a wall after being captured at gunpoint by Russian soldiers. Good old *Boys' Own* adventures. Just what I had always dreamed of doing. Plaudit followed plaudit. My career was on track, and the track was golden.

Imagine my state of mind in 1981. I had landed the plum job at ITN, against all expectations. There could not have been a more exciting time to take up the Washington posting, with a new President in the White House. It was mine, all mine. On the personal level, I was leaving behind that beautiful and gorgeous woman I had been secretly in love with for almost a decade, and whom I had kissed in one unforgettable moment in the pouring rain. But she had given me hope by saying she would try to get over to the US to visit her family, and if she did maybe we could see each other.

We're down in France. Bon loves it here so much. She gets gently confused, though. This morning when I brought tea up to bed, she had already dressed. I have learned not to snap now. So I quietly said, Take your clothes off and get back into bed, then after tea you can shower. She said yes, I didn't need to get dressed.

She went into the bathroom and I listened at the door. She was whispering to herself, 'Right, clothes off and then I shower. OK. Right, take my clothes off first … now shower.' It was quite a relief when I heard the water come on.

That remark Bonnie had made, albeit a year or more before, about how sad it was that I wasn't seeing my parents, had simmered in me. What I was doing to my 'old' family, was wrong, plain wrong, and I *had* to do something about it.

In July 1981, days before leaving for the US, I braced myself and made a journey. I invented an excuse for leaving the house a couple of hours earlier than usual ('need to sort stuff out in the office') and travelled up to London. Instead of going straight to the ITN office, I stopped off in Baker Street. Heart pounding, I entered the large block of flats immediately over the tube station, the block where I had grown up. Where my parents lived. There was a porter behind the desk, quite elderly. I recognised him. He smiled broadly when he saw me. 'Hello, Mr John. It's been a while. You'll find them upstairs. Second floor. They'll be so pleased to see you.' I nodded, couldn't say anything, throat closed up.

I walked along the corridor, the sights, sounds, smells of my childhood invading and battering my senses. I stood outside their door, paused, fought back tears, breathed deeply to steady myself, and rang the bell. A woman I didn't recognise answered the door. She looked at me, frowned, then gasped, her hand flying to her mouth. 'There, in the kitchen,' she said in a foreign accent, pointing to her left.

I walked to the back of the entrance hall and took the few short steps to the kitchen. Then I saw them. Mum was sitting at the kitchen table, Dad was standing behind her, his hands on her shoulders. Their mouths opened, shock in their eyes, bewilderment on their faces. I opened my mouth to speak, but nothing came out. My eyes filled up. Mum leapt out of the chair and flung her arms round me. I cried into her neck. Finally I looked at Dad. He had tears in his eyes, and a false-angry look on his face. 'About bloody time,' he said, or words to that effect. 'Come on down to the sitting room.'

We sat and talked and talked and talked. Just one or two things to catch up on. Like several years, and three grandchildren. I gave them photos of the boys I'd secretly had printed. The years melted away. I couldn't stay for long. I had to go in to work. I told them I was sorry from the bottom of my heart for what I had done to them, and that I would make it right again. I would be in Washington for four years, I said, but I would stay in touch, albeit surreptitiously, and one day, not far off, everything would be normal again.

They hugged me till I thought I would burst. It was the Prodigal Son. If Dad could have killed a fatted calf, he would have.

I didn't tell them about Bonnie, because I could see no way of making my dream come true. Nor did I tell them that if it hadn't been for her passionate remark, and the power of that kiss, I wouldn't have had the strength to do what I had done that day. A shameful admission, but true.

I was at the computer just now. Bon came in and recited her full name – first name, middle, then surname. She smiled at me in triumph. Before I could stop myself, I said yes, that's right, but why did you say it? Because it's true, she said, raising her fists in triumph. This is the woman who 10 years ago taught me how to use the computer, and almost 30 years ago was responsible for my long overdue reunion with my parents.

Things in Washington began well enough. I filed reports for *News at Ten* from around the US. Mostly they were 'soft' items, as Americans redis-covered their pride after President Carter's disastrous handling of the Iran crisis. Ronald Reagan told his people they were not to blame, there was nothing morally superior about Islam, and in his State of the Union address in 1982 he memorably defined the Soviet Union as the 'evil empire'. Nobody had stood up to Communism like that before. We were not to know it, but it was the beginning of the process that would culminate seven years later with the destruction of the Berlin Wall and the fall of Communism. President Reagan had been right.

But something strange was happening to me. I was not settling happily into my role as US correspondent. I found the 'soft' stories, *Look at Life* stories as I dismissively called them, difficult, and when it came to political stories in Washington, I was struggling. With hindsight, I can see it clearly (in fact, I saw it clearly just a few years later): I was a 'fireman', it was what I had always wanted to be, and I had proved to be quite good at it. What I was not good at was unearthing stories, finding them, tracking them down. Give me a plane crash, a sudden disaster, a war, you name it, and I was in my element – get there fast, turn out report after report, come home. There was another kind of story I was also proving to be less than good at: politics. I was not, never have been, and still am not, a networker. Not for me the working lunch with contacts, probing them discreetly, getting the inside story. I had very little interest in the workings of Capitol Hill – not ideal for a US correspondent. I can state all this now, but at the time it was not quite as glaringly obvious. Me? Not good at something? Don't be ridiculous, it must be the something that is at fault.

One further fact increased my unease. My opposite number, the BBC's US correspondent – against whose work mine would be judged – happened to be one of the best of our generation, he of the white suit, the future Independent MP Martin Bell. Martin had already outgunned me once, covering the handover of independence to the Central American country of Belize. While I attempted to follow Princess Michael of Kent's official schooner to an offshore island, by hiring a rickety boat with two outboard motors, one of which broke down, leaving my crew and me stranded, Martin filed a comprehensive report on the state of Belize's economy.

I sensed that all was not right. I was given to understand, subtly but to the point, that there were rumblings in London that maybe I was not up to the job. I wasn't fazed. Hell, I would ride it out. A good strong story or two and they would see what I was made of. But I was about to be found out.

On 2nd April 1982, Argentine forces invaded and occupied the Falkland Islands and South Georgia. From out of nowhere, Britain was on the brink of war. The United States administration took it upon itself to lead diplomatic attempts to prevent conflict, in the shape of Secretary of State Alexander Haig. He undertook a triangular diplomatic shuttle between Washington, London and Buenos Aires. The London end was covered by our political editor, a senior reporter was dispatched to Buenos Aires, and it fell to me to cover the Washington angle. This involved attending regular press conferences at the State Department, as well as off-the-record briefings by the British ambassador, Sir Nicholas Henderson, at the British Embassy.

At the State Department I was not asking the right questions, and my reports failed to capture the nuances of America's negotiating tactics. My understanding of the subtleties offered to us at the ambassador's briefings escaped me. So came the word from the foreign desk in London. One day the phone in the office rang and on the line was David Nicholas. The top man. The boss. 'Are you properly plumbed in to Capitol Hill?' he asked. 'Of course, David,' I replied. 'Then tell me which senators you are speaking to. Who is briefing you? Who are you having lunch with?' 'Er ...'

Still I was not overly concerned. Can you believe that? It would still come right, I was convinced. My posting was for four years. These were early days.

Then something happened that was to take my mind thoroughly off work-related matters. I heard from Bonnie that she was coming to the US to visit her family in New Jersey.

* * * *

It is a cold wet Easter Saturday afternoon down in France and we have just watched the 1960s film *55 Days At Peking* on the television, starring Charlton Heston as the hard-as-nails heroic American major and David Niven as the suave, cool and stiff-upper-lipped British ambassador. In real life, one died of Alzheimer's, the other of motor neurone disease. Once you get caught up in the dreadful subject of brain disease, you tend to be aware of things like that.

It is getting dark by the time the film finishes. I say I will pull the curtains in the *séjour*. Good idea, Bon says, I will help you. Then into the kitchen to empty the dishwasher. A few minutes later she goes into the *séjour* and opens the curtains. I say nothing, but when the dishwasher is empty I say, gosh, it's dark and wet, I'll pull the *séjour* curtains. Good idea, she says. We do them again together. A few minutes later she goes back into the *séjour* and opens them.

I see the funny side and give her a big hug. She doesn't know why she has deserved this, but she smiles.

* * * *

It was all I could think of. I had to see her. I *had* to. I called her at home in the UK when I knew her husband would be at work. She said of course she would see me – that was why she was coming over! I was shocked. Final proof. It wouldn't be easy, and it couldn't be for long, she said, but somehow she would make it happen.

On a day in the summer of 1982, I met her for lunch in Washington. We threw ourselves at each other, kissed, embraced, hugged. It was slightly early, so we were able to find a quiet table in the corner of a small Italian restaurant. We sat and started talking, and talked and talked and talked. The *maître d'* came to take our order again, again and again, raising his shoulders in Italian exasperation. Still we talked. *Prego, signor e signore?* We muttered something to him. We barely ate. So many plans, so many possibilities, all completely hopeless. I kept my hand on hers, just wanted to touch her, not let her go. In between the torrent of whispered words, a bite or two of food. *Dolci, signor e signore?* A shake of the head, and still the words flowed. I looked her in the eye, stroked her cheek.

She told me more about her life at home. Her husband was not entirely the attentive soul he appeared to be. She didn't have a lot to complain about except that his life revolved around work and he didn't share it with her, leaving her to raise their sons and clean the house. She felt neglected, lonely. 'That night you kissed me,' she said, 'I knew my marriage was over.' Stunned? I was struck dumb. But how to be together, Bonnie and me? That was the question we asked again and again, but could not answer. On and on we talked, trying to work out if there was a way we could have a future together.

Finally we were brought sharply back to planet earth. The Italian boss, standing facing us, shoulders raised, arms outstretched, palms toward us, behind him an empty restaurant. 'Eh,' he said, 'this is a-love, not a-minestrone.' We both dissolved in laughter.

I had an office to go back to, Bon had a train to catch. We said goodbye rather perfunctorily outside the restaurant. 'I must see you again,' I said. She nodded. A flash of light in my head. 'New York,' I said. 'Can you come to New York? I can invent a story in New York. There's always something happening up there. Could you come over again?' She looked worried. 'I don't know. I'll need to think of how. I'll let you know.' And she was gone.

What was I doing? Back in our rented house, the atmosphere was worsening. There had been a change in my attitude, brought about by several factors. We were away from the family house in Henley, the house where the boys had grown up, and I had no emotional ties to the house we were now in. The reunion with my parents had underlined for me how wrong I had been to allow the rift to happen – and how wrong Moya had been to ask me to cut all contact with them in the first place. There had been 'The Kiss', and now Bonnie – woman of my dreams for so long – was telling me candidly she wanted to be with me every day, night and day. I was emboldened, empowered.

A few months after that lunch with Bonnie in Washington, I saw a story in the US press that British holidaymakers were coming over to New York on shopping trips because of the strength of sterling and also the relative cheapness of American goods. Perfect story, I thought. I sent a telex to the foreign desk in London proposing a major report, a potential lead to part two of *News at Ten*, filming Brits shopping on Fifth Avenue – cameras, CD players, even clothes in the big stores like Macy's and Saks Fifth Avenue. It would, I wrote, mean a full day's filming with a two-night stay in New York.

The reply wasn't good. The foreign editor felt the story wasn't strong enough to merit such a trip. If there were two or three other stories to mop up at the same time, maybe. But on its own, no. If I was keen to do it, though, why not a swift day trip to New York – surely all the filming necessary could be accomplished in two to three hours?

This was, of course, journalistically absolutely the right response. It just happened to be not the response I wanted. But why should I allow that to deter me? I was more concerned with affairs of the heart, of considerably greater importance than any journalistic consideration. I looked at the diary. I ringed three days the following week. I phoned Bon in Henley and gave her the dates. I implored her to fly over. Invent something, I said, anything, only just be in New York for these dates. She sounded flustered. She had her boys to think of, then aged 14 and 11. She would have to think of something to tell her husband. I pushed her. What better chance would we ever have? She told me she would do all she could, but it would be difficult.

On the appointed date, I flew to New York. I was, quite simply, committing slow but certain professional suicide.

✻ ✻ ✻ ✻

Humour. That's the thing. Usual difficulty getting Bon to take her clothes off to shower after breakfast. 'Why must I? Why have I got to do this?' I said 'It's a small price to pay for being beautiful.' A beatific smile spread over her face and she co-operated fully.

* * * *

She had made it possible. I gave her the name of the hotel – the Harley on East 42nd Street – and told her I would be there from 6pm. She told me she would try to get there as soon after that as possible.

It was a beautiful room, with lush furnishings and a luxurious king-size bed. I fussed around, making sure everything was perfect. Beautiful soft towelling dressing gowns, his and hers, towels you could wrap round yourself twice, large bath and spacious walk-in shower. It was perfect. I rang room service and ordered a bottle of champagne. It arrived before she did, which I was pleased about.

The phone rang. 'I'm in the lobby.' As calmly as I could, I gave her the room number. My heart was pounding, my skin tingling. I forced myself to count slowly to 20, then went to the door and held it open. I listened for the lift doors opening. Nothing. I waited, my breathing becoming shallower. Still nothing. I cast my eyes back into the room to check for the umpteenth time that everything was in order. Suddenly a flurry of movement, the sound of quick breathing, the rustle of clothes. In a flash, head down, she brushed past me into the room.

Her face was flushed, her eyes wide. I put my hands on her shoulders to steady her. 'Are you all right?' She nodded, and slowly her breathing calmed down. 'God, what an experience.' 'What do you mean?' 'As soon as I walked into the lobby, I saw this man looking at me. Had a pass or something round his neck, so I knew he was security. After I phoned you, he walked over to me. I knew what he was thinking. He asked me if I was a guest. I said no, but I was coming to visit a friend. From England. He looked as if he was going to question me further. But then he nodded and walked away.' 'My God,' I said. She nodded quickly. 'He thought I was a hooker.' She looked alarmed, I looked alarmed, then we both dissolved into laughter.

She was wearing a dark pink suede suit, with a plain mauve blouse underneath. That suit was one of my favourites, and I had told her so when she had worn it to a fancy do we had been to with our spouses in London. That's why I wore it, she said, because I knew you liked it. I sat her on the end of the bed, put my arms round her, and kissed her. She responded instantly. Gently I laid her back on the bed, opened the suit jacket, and kissed her again, more softly this time.

I opened the champagne and poured two glasses. 'A toast,' I said. 'To our future together. Lord knows how we'll achieve it, but we'll do it somehow.' We clinked our glasses and drank. Later I ordered dinner from room service.

I remember now that we didn't talk much that evening. What was there to say? We could go through all the impossible dreams and ideas again, as we had at that Italian restaurant in Washington, but where would it get us? There was another reason for our silence – well, mine at any rate. I knew we were together, and were going to be together for the next two nights. I wanted nothing to intrude on that delicious thought.

It came time for bed. 'You get into bed,' she said, 'and I'll join you in a few moments.' She went into the bathroom. When she emerged she was wearing a white towelling robe. I had dimmed the lights. She stood by the side of the bed, fixed her eyes on mine, unbelted the robe and let it fall from her shoulders. She climbed into the bed.

* * * *

Ah, my Bonnie, I remember it as if it were yesterday, every sensation, every glorious moment, the little pulsating sounds you made, the gentle smile on your upturned lips. You make that sound now, quite often, but there is distress in it. You made it when I got you ready for bed last night, didn't you? You hate having to take your clothes off to get into your nightie, you ask me why do I have to do this, and you make despairing little sobbing sounds. They go into me like a thousand sharp needles. I try to reassure you, but know I am making you unhappy, and that hurts. Me, making my Bonnie unhappy? How could it have come to this? But once you're in your nightie you're fine, you even thank me.

So off we go to the bathroom. I hand you your toothbrush and you start to brush your teeth. Damn, how could I have been so stupid? I take it gently from you and put toothpaste on it. You let me, you're not angry. All the time I am saying reassuring things. You let me help you, even with the most intimate things. In fact, you're grateful. Thank God. I couldn't handle it if you kept getting angry with me.

I tuck you into bed like a caring parent. I return to the bathroom, content to have just a minute or two on my own. Last night I looked at myself long and hard in the mirror. Sad face. John the lover now John the carer. I force a theatrical smile. Make it as wide as I can. God it makes me look stupid, but it makes me laugh for a moment. I get into bed and we have a peck of a goodnight kiss. As always, my mind starts to roll back the years, but fortunately I am asleep before I become too miserable.

I cursed myself for having wasted five hours sleeping in that hotel room. Five hours of unconsciousness. Stupid boy! I wake you gently, and without opening your eyes you are smiling and we are joined again, from our lips down to our toes.

You get up and make me a cup of tea. I remember you walked across the end of the bed. You wore the towelling robe, and on your head was a white towelling turban. You turned to me and you were smiling. 'I must look silly,' you said. Silly? *Silly?* I had never seen anything so beautiful in my life.

We lingered over breakfast in the room and I reluctantly began to turn my attention to the day's filming. I had a story to shoot. I knew I could knock it off in a couple of hours and get back to the hotel. As I left the room, I turned back for a last look. Bon was sitting up in bed, still in the robe and turban. It took me a moment to realise that what I thought was a towel she was holding to her face was, in fact, the shirt I had been wearing the day before.

I linked up with my camera crew and explained that we would have a trawl down Fifth Avenue and film Brits shopping. My cameraman asked me what stores I had arranged this with. I said I hadn't made any prior arrangements, we would just suck it and see. He raised an eyebrow. It won't be that straightforward, he said. You can't just walk in with cameras and expect to start filming. I told him not to be silly. This was America. You could film anything you liked, anywhere you liked.

Turned out he was right. By lunchtime we hadn't shot a foot of film. Never mind, let's go to one of the electronic shops. That's where we'll find the Brits. We found the shop all right, but the moment we walked in with our camera gear the manager came straight over waving his hands. You can't film in here, he said. What was going on, I wondered? He explained that the shop had a strict policy of privacy towards its customers – we couldn't film anyone in the act of buying. I protested – free country, free press, what if the customer agreed, and so on. Ever tried arguing with a New Yorker? Doesn't work.

I was beginning to get just the inklings of a certain feeling of anxiety. My arguing turned to pleading. Finally the manager made a small concession. We could film the goods in the shop, as long as we did not identify the shop, and he would give me an interview saying that he had noticed an increase in British shoppers in the previous few weeks. Phew, I thought, at least that will give me a story.

By late afternoon that was all we had. Not much of a story, said my cameraman. I was satisfied. I knew we had enough. We shot some footage of anonymous people window shopping, walking in and out of the big stores. I added a piece to camera, me strolling along Fifth Avenue saying how Brits were taking advantage of the strong pound and the lower prices here, making it worth coming to shop in New York even with the cost of an airfare. By six o'clock I was back in the Harley with my Bonnie.

That evening I said I wanted to take her out to dinner. She wore a dark chiffon dress with large colourful flowers, belted at the waist, pleated at the front. Another of my favourites. Under it, oh yes, stockings and suspenders. Naturally. Those cream combs held back her lovely hair. I smiled when I saw them. I knew you would like that, she said. Had I ever been happier? I don't think so.

I took her by the arm and walked her to a restaurant I knew. The manager sat us at a table in the window with Bon facing out to the street and me facing into the restaurant. The cold air was coming through the glass, and so we moved to a table further in. The manager came over, arms out, and asked in a voice that passes for polite in New York, 'So what did you do that for?' I said defensively, 'Er, it's a little cold by the window. It's warmer here. Is that ok?' 'So now the pretty lady cannot be seen from the street. Sheesh!' and he walked away in disgust. He'd wanted her to be seen from the street because it would be good for business!

I laughed out loud and she laughed in an embarrassed way. For many years thereafter, whenever we went into a restaurant, I would imitate that manager in an exaggerated New York accent.

The next morning had to come, there was no way of stopping it. I wanted divine powers so that I could make time stand still. Sadly my urgent pleas with any deity there might be up there went unanswered.

Breakfast in the room the next morning was a subdued affair. I can remember exactly what I said to her. 'We've lived together for the last two days. I know what it is like now to live with you. It's what I want for the rest of my life. This is a turning point. After New York things can never be the same for me.' She looked at me with a serious face. 'It's what I want too,' she said.

As for my ace report on Brits shopping in New York, I satellited it to London but it never made *News at Ten*. The foreign editor told me it was one of the weakest pieces he had ever seen. Still I didn't see the warning signs.

* * * *

I get up from the breakfast table and walk across the kitchen to the cupboards, instantly forgetting why.

'What have I come here for?' Silence. 'Why have I come here, my Bonnie?'

'I don't know, and I don't care.'

Her words sting. 'Oh darling, don't say that. It hurts.'

'Well, everyone else is doing it, so why shouldn't I?'

* * * *

We spoke transatlantically several times over the coming months, often for two hours or more. Finally we made a pact. We would both tell our spouses we were leaving them.

We knew that what we were doing was wrong. We were married, me with three boys, she with two. We were breaking up our families. There would be hurt and pain. Morally it was indefensible. But we could not be stopped. It sounds melodramatic, and I can hardly believe I am about to write a sentence more suited to a bodice-ripping novel. We truly could no longer imagine life without each other.

Life with Bonnie, I knew, would be calm. I had known it for a long time: the New York sojourn simply confirmed it. I knew something else too. It would be very different to the life I was currently living with my wife. Bonnie was even-tempered, wise and kind. Where Moya and I seemed to disagree on everything, in the short time Bonnie and I had spent together we discovered that we liked *exactly* the same things, in whatever field. There were no arguments. I also found, to my obvious delight, that if I expressed an opinion on whatever subject, Bonnie would nod and agree. It was not something I was used to, and I liked it.

Relations between Moya and me were worsening, our differences becoming more pronounced, not least because I was being slightly less acquiescent. There were other reasons. She'd wanted me to take the Washington posting, yet once we were there she wasn't happy. The ITN house, which we had visited a couple of months before on a familiarisation trip and which she had liked very much, was now suddenly unacceptable and she insisted that we move. My bosses at ITN were a bit shocked. She picked holes in everything I did, anything I said, and I no longer gave in quite so easily, which didn't help.

Bonnie had given me a little present in New York, a small book with deep red velvet covers entitled *Love: a celebration*. It was an anthology of love poems. Inside she had written, 'For my Poodle, with all my love Bonnie'. The book is sitting alongside my laptop now. In January 1983, there was a massive snowfall in Washington and I couldn't get home. I stayed the night in the Mayflower Hotel. I had the little book with me. I read the poems. One, in particular, I read again and again and again. It was by D.H. Lawrence and it was entitled 'All I Ask'.

'All I ask of a woman is that she feel gently towards me
when my heart feels kindly towards her,
and there shall be the soft, soft tremor as of unheard bells between us.
It is all I ask.
I am so tired of violent women lashing out
and insisting on being loved, when there is
no love in them.'

Shortly after this, Moya and I had the grand-daddy of all rows, the one that marked the end. It began with a classic domestic, a kind of *Who's Afraid of Virginia Wolf?* without the other couple, and it ended with us both realising that the marriage was over. Things had been said and done from which there was no way back any more.

On Sunday 13th February 1983, with the help of my cameraman and his van, I moved out of the large house rented by ITN in a suburb of Washington DC and into a bedsit near Rockville Park close to the centre of the city.

Lying in bed this morning, Bon said something. I asked, 'What did you say?' She said 'I don't know but I'll know by next year.' We both dissolved in giggles.

Bonnie said she wouldn't be able to come over to join me until late April. There was no question of her bringing the boys because she didn't want to disrupt their schooling at a crucial stage when I would be in Washington for only a limited time anyway. She had to sort out their school arrangements, clothes, all the normal domestic things she would be leaving behind. I told her how sorry I was she was having to go through all that, but she said that at least her husband was behaving very reasonably, given the circumstances. He was hardly happy that his wife was about to leave him, but he told her he would not stand in her way or make things unnecessarily difficult.

Late April was more than two months away. I am not by nature a patient person, but I put myself through a self-designed patience course. When taking the escalator at my local metro station, I forced myself to stay still and wait until my feet reached the step-off point at the very top before moving. In the street I slowed my pace just a notch. When eating I chewed each mouthful that little bit longer. In short, every activity I performed, I tried to make it take a little more time. That way, I felt, the two months or so might seem slightly less long.

Then something came to my rescue – at least, that was how it felt. The Queen and Duke of Edinburgh were to make a tour of the west coast of America. Surprisingly, during 30 years on the throne and dozens of official visits the world over, the Queen had never visited California. It was announced that in March they would more than rectify this, starting in San Diego in southern California, going right up the coast and across the border into Canada, ending the tour in Vancouver.

By now, even with my mind focused on other matters, I was coming to realise that my reputation as ace correspondent was taking something of a battering in London. A colleague back in the newsroom tipped me off that the knives were out. It was worrying, of course, but I *still* failed to appreciate the gravity of it, even when I was told that those wielding the knives were pretty senior figures. I knew I had a four-year contract, all right maybe I was going through a bit of a trough, but one good story and hey, all would be right again. The royal visit to the west coast was heaven-sent.

It began badly and got worse. I can't now remember what the content of the first report I satellited to London was, but I do remember the foreign editor telling me it was considered transmittable on *News at Ten* only after some major re-editing in London. The high point of the visit was to be the arrival of the royal couple in Los Angeles. The plan was for them to arrive by boat, accompanied by a flotilla, and to be greeted with fanfare by President Reagan and First Lady Nancy as they stepped ashore.

The problem, though, was that a day earlier a storm had blown up, the rain came down in torrents, the sea became dark and treacherous, and the forecast was of no let-up for days. There was a hasty rescheduling of events, with the royal arrival now happening in the rather less spectacular form of a motorcade. I shrugged this off and filed a standard report, pointing out the change of plan, but focusing on what was planned for the Queen and Duke – walkabouts, a visit to Hollywood, a banquet hosted by the Reagans, Frank Sinatra to sing for the Queen, British actors and actresses based in Hollywood to meet her, and so on. All in all, I thought I had done a pretty good job.

London did not agree. The BBC report – Martin Bell, of course – had been superb, I was told. Graphic footage of raging seas and tossing boats, people dashing for cover through a biblical downpour, stunned locals saying they had never seen anything like it, flustered officials struggling to reschedule everything at the last minute – and this was California in the spring! I was ordered to do a swift catch-up report, with a warning that much better coverage was expected from me.

Did I take this to heart and buck up my ideas? Judge for yourself. I attended a banquet to which I received a personal invitation. It said *President and Mrs Ronald Reagan, and guests of honour Her Majesty Queen Elizabeth and His Royal Highness the Duke of Edinburgh, request the company of John Suchet at a banquet ...* Well, you would go too, wouldn't you? In the presentation line I met the legendary Alistair Cooke, journalist and broadcaster famed for his *Letter from America* on BBC radio. When I reached the royal couple, the Queen proffered a tiny gloved hand in such a way that I only grasped the tips of her fingers. Expecting the Duke to be something of a 'man's man', I gave him a knowing smile and pointed out I was a journalist. He took my hand, and in one swift movement I found myself several feet away. So that's how they do it, I thought.

The evening went well. I snatched a quick 'on the hoof' couple of words with Frank Sinatra, I interviewed a young Anthony Hopkins trying to make a name for himself in Hollywood, Julie Andrews gave me a smile that would have melted an iceberg and answered my fawning questions graciously, and even an 87-year-old George Burns did a comic turn for me. I basked in what was really rather an exciting occasion for a journalist, forgetting the golden rule that a good journalist will observe, rather than participate. My report made *News at Ten*, but won no plaudits.

Have I finished my tale of woe, you ask? Oh dear me no. British officials briefed me that the Queen and Duke were to be guests of the Reagans at their ranch in the Californian hills, and asked me if I would like a place with my camera crew on the press bus. Of course I said yes. I did not change my mind, even when the kindly Martin Bell (perhaps sensing I needed a bit of guidance) advised me not to go. You'll be out of touch for hours, he said. Better to stay in Los Angeles and take coverage from American TV. He was right, of course. Sure, I got excellent coverage of the Queen and President Reagan riding horses in torrential rain, of the two couples posing for the cameras again in a downpour, and even picked up the sound of Nancy prompting her husband when a question was thrown by a reporter (not me). I knew I had enough for a good piece.

So had Martin. Just as good as me, and he had stayed at base and filmed a lot of other material to give his report more breadth and gravitas. (Shades of Belize.) I was thoroughly bested again.

All right. I shall spare you any more self-inflicted humiliation. By the end of the trip, my bosses in London had more or less given up on me. I was pretty much a lost cause. On a personal level, it was even worse. The continual rain and cold temperatures had got to me. By the time I reached Vancouver, I had a nasty cough, which I could not shake. When I breathed deeply, fluid rattled in my lungs. This had not happened to me before. I went to see a doctor. At first he thought I might have contracted pneumonia. In the event, he diagnosed bronchitis. I was slightly hurt when I was offered not an ounce of sympathy from London.

If I had any doubt that my stock had plummeted, it was settled once and for all when a senior foreign desk journalist announced he was coming to Washington and wanted to see me. In the office he sat me down and explained that the editor-in-chief, David Nicholas, was seriously worried about me. What had happened? My reports were shocking. Why? In mitigation I explained what had happened to me on the domestic front. It must have affected my journalistic judgment, I said. He said my marital problems were an open secret in London, but that was no excuse for unprofessionalism. I was United States correspondent, for God's sake, and things were expected of me. Finally he hinted darkly that if my work didn't improve, action would have to be taken. He didn't elucidate and I didn't probe.

On my own in my bedsit, with weeks still to go until Bonnie's arrival, I pondered my position. My career, I finally acknowledged, was in trouble. I had been given the biggest reporter's job in ITN's gift, and it appeared I had blown it. What did the future hold for me professionally? I had no idea, but it was not looking good.

How bad did I feel about this? How worried was I? This may shock you, but really I was not all that concerned. Why not? Because soon my Bonnie would be with me. Soon my new life would begin.

We fly back from France and at Stansted use the moving walkway. I go ahead and come off first. Mistake. Bonnie is wandering from side to side on it, lost. A man pulling a suitcase pushes angrily past. I try to gesture. Another pushes past, jostling Bon and making her distressed. As he walks angrily off, he says, 'You're supposed to stand on the right'.

I feel a surge of anger. I want to shout, 'My wife has dementia, you idiot.' Instead I say, 'Fuck off'. Even as I say it, I know I shouldn't. I should just take Bon by the arm and calm her down. I hope he doesn't turn round and start a scene. He doesn't. He is in too much of a hurry. Good. I must learn to stay calm, whatever. My priority is Bon, not getting my own back on some idiot.

✳ ✳ ✳ ✳

I was living the life of a bachelor and finding it quite a challenge, albeit a rather enjoyable one. Breakfast was a boiled egg and a cup of tea, and in the evening I cooked myself a leg of chicken with frozen spinach. To vary it, I would cook chicken breast with frozen peas. Occasionally I bought pork, but it was a bit bland. I tried to cook steak but always overdid it.

I didn't mind having confined surroundings. I am by nature tidy and the few clothes I had brought with me were neatly stacked on shelves. It reminded me of my university days. I set up the old manual typewriter Mum and Dad had given me for my 17th birthday, and which had now been round the world with me, and typed page after page of my longing for Bonnie and the joy that I knew lay ahead. (You are spared – I have long since shredded it.)

There was, inevitably, a cloud. I wasn't seeing my boys. I saw Rory once – we went 10-pin bowling on one of those difficult single-parent outings. Kieran was at school in Maryland, Damian at boarding school back in the UK. I spoke to Moya several times on the phone in an effort to see the boys, but her response was always that they didn't want to see me. I know now that was untrue, though of course I didn't know it at the time. Fair enough, I thought, I had left the marital home, made their mother unhappy, and left them without a dad in the house. I knew they would need time and that I shouldn't force things. In the end, I was sure it would turn out all right. (Just as I had felt over my parents. I should have known better.)

One Sunday morning I went across the road to a café and ordered a coffee. A disheveled man sat at the counter next to me. Bearded, shabbily dressed, baggy eyes half-closed from a no-doubt sleepless night, in typical American fashion he opened conversation with me. I scarcely listened to his drawl, and he finally gave up. He looked like a man who had recently left his wife and set up in a bedsit somewhere. Why would I want to talk to him?

✳ ✳ ✳ ✳

An utterly traumatic 24 hours. As I write this, in mid April 2009, I realise it is 26 years minus one week, my Bonnie, since you flew to America and we began our new lives. Yesterday we went to the christening of your granddaughter, your son Hereward's daughter. As a christening present, we took her a beautiful emerald ring, the ring I bought you for your 60th birthday. How you loved it! It sparkled on your finger, catching the sparkle in your eyes. You wore it to so many special occasions. I took it out when you were getting ready for the RTS awards ceremony last year when they made that dreadful mistake and gave me the piece of engraved glass. You said what a lovely ring. I asked if you could remember when I had given it to you, but you shook your head and smiled. I mentally smacked myself for asking. I tried to fit it on your finger, but it wouldn't go over the first joint. I stifled my disappointment, said never mind, and hastily put it back. You didn't seem concerned. So then I thought why not pass it on to your granddaughter? Keep it in the family.

Your ex-husband was at the christening, naturally, since he is grandfather. He pecks you on the cheek, you smile, but I don't see recognition on your face. Later, ironically, it is he who drives us to the station. You get another couple of pecks, I get a cursory handshake (he is hardly going to treat me like a long-lost buddy) and we walk to the platform. I know I shouldn't ask you this, but as nonchalantly as I can I say, 'Did you recognise that chap, the man who drove us to the station?' You say, 'No'. I don't say anything more.

In bed later I lie awake for some time, profoundly depressed. You didn't recognise the man to whom you were married for the best part of 20 years, with whom you had two children. It didn't worry you. You showed no distress during the whole day, although I know that your son, your grandchildren, other members of the family were lost on you. It has made me realise that if I were to go away for, say, a month, maybe two, you would probably forget who I am. This has been the strongest evidence yet of what this dreadful disease is doing to your memory, and I shudder at the thought of what stage it will be at in a year's time, or less. But in a curious way I am calm. The big issues seem almost easier to cope with than the minor ones.

This was concrete evidence, undeniable, unambiguous. I feel so sorry for you, it is impossible not to become tearful. These words I am typing are shimmering through a tearful veil. It makes me all the more determined to be patient with the smaller issues, the minor eccentricities that are part of the same affliction and not just some bloody-mindedness on your part.

I shall return now to writing about the glorious past, when so much lay ahead of us, so much seemed possible. That'll cheer me up. Maybe.

＊ ＊ ＊ ＊

I like Billy Joel's songs. There, that's a cheery thought. I was in my bedsit one evening when up came his latest on the small TV. It was called 'Uptown Girl'. The video showed the model Christie Brinkley pulling into a petrol station in her chauffeur-driven limo, stepping out and shimmying arrogantly across the forecourt in swaying summer dress, killer stilettos and wide-brimmed hat, pursued by a gang of oil-stained mechanics led by Billy Joel, half crouching as they trailed in her wake, clicking their fingers as he sang about his 'Uptown Girl'.

I yelped with recognition. Ms Brinkley, blonde, pale-skinned, beautiful, smiling seductively, the arrogance an act, pursued by olive-skinned, dark-haired Joel in an impossible bid to gain her attention. At the end, of course, she climbs onto his motorbike and off they ride together, her hat in her hands and her long hair waving in the wind. It was Bonnie and me.

A few weeks ago, I downloaded that video onto my laptop and watched it for first time in 26 years, headphones clasped to my ears. Oh boy, did the tears run down my face. There, all depressed again.

The date was set. She said she was flying over on 27th April.

I informed London I wanted to take a week's holiday in early May and booked a small apartment on the seashore in South Carolina. On the morning of the 27th, I picked her up at Baltimore Washington International and drove her back to my bedsit. She did that twirl, and I knew our lives would never be the same again. We were at last together.

Chapter 3

I am an amateur photographer. My grandfather was a professional – a Fleet Street photographer for 50 years. In a way I have followed him professionally, and like him I always have a small camera at the ready. My photographs are not arty – my brother David is the one for that – but they capture the moment. (Recently, at a family reunion, David ran around with his super-slick camera missing all the shots while he set the focus, aperture, timer, this and that, in between gulps of wine, crying 'Missed it' every time he pressed the shutter, while I captured every moment, albeit out of focus and poorly framed.)

The purpose of relating this is to help you understand why I took that photograph of Bonnie and me at our first dinner in the bedsit, and why there are so many photographs of her in this book. From the moment she joined me, I made up my mind to chronicle our life together, from the beginning to the end. And, being a great planner, I thought I knew exactly what the end would be.

In our early days together, I told her I would fill album after album, and then in our extreme old age, probably in a care home, we would turn the pages of the albums together, and remember. Yes! she would exclaim joyfully. In the years that followed, she never minded me whipping the camera out. I rarely needed to ask her to pose. Each camera I've had clearly fell in love with her; no camera is capable of taking a poor picture of her.

I kept my word. I filled album after album. Only in recent years have I stopped, because it became clear that the illness was preventing her from enjoying the pictures. Instead of an album, I now put pictures digitally on a picture frame, so they are running the whole time – the family, children and grandchildren, us. But she doesn't look at them. I think it's a defensive mechanism on her part, to avoid having to try to remember who the pictures are of. I occasionally draw her attention to one, mentioning the name, but she just smiles without saying anything.

So far in writing this book I have used just my memory. That picture of the first dinner has been on my laptop for years. Now I am about to write about South Carolina, and that means going to Album Number One. More tears.

South Carolina, ah South Carolina. Isle of Palms, to be precise, a short distance east of Charleston. Our private domain, our little corner of paradise. It has faded from your mind now, my darling, but to me, well, if I close my eyes tight I can *smell* it.

You on the beach, you in the sea, you at the cooker, you relaxing on the sofa. I couldn't take my eyes off you. You insisted on taking the occasional picture of me. I didn't know my face was capable of smiling so wide, the corners of my lips reaching halfway round my head. Oh boy, was I happy.

We went to bed together, woke up together, ate together, laughed together. We were a couple. With every passing hour, I learned more about you – what you thought, what you believed, what you read, what you liked. I told you I liked big modern American novels – John Steinbeck in particular, James Jones, Herman Wouk. So did you. You said you loved history, the American Civil War, the history of the Deep South. I said I did too. I said I wasn't religious; in fact, I found organised religion with its bizarre rituals and ridiculous rules about what you could eat and couldn't eat, absurd and even dangerous. You agreed. At one point, as nonchalantly as possible I asked, 'Who is your favourite composer?' You thought for a moment. 'I think it has to be Beethoven,' you said. It wouldn't have mattered if you had said Stockhausen, but you didn't, you said Beethoven. I told you that I had listened to Beethoven endlessly in the difficult weeks before I left Moya, the *Eroica Symphony* in particular. You told me your favourite Beethoven was the *Pastoral Symphony*, but you asked me to teach you the *Eroica*, tell you how Beethoven had come to compose it, what it meant, what to listen out for. I thrilled to hear that. No one had ever asked me to teach them anything about art before. (I couldn't have known just what a meeting of minds it was, given that I was to go on and write five books about Beethoven, all with Bonnie's endless encouragement.)

And so I explored your mind. Of course, I explored you in other ways too, and you encouraged me. I had never been so happy.

We spent a day in Charleston. We had lunch in a balcony restaurant in an old antebellum building. I took pictures of you at the table. A Dutch couple at the next table couldn't help smiling as I took picture after picture, my face beaming happiness from every pore. 'Here,' said the man, 'let me take a picture of both of you. That's what you really need.' The picture he took shows two people totally in love, with not a care in the world.

The week soon came to an end, and if there had been no care in the world down in South Carolina, that was not the case back in Washington. I filed the occasional story, with no encouragement from London. Then, on 18th June, the space shuttle *Challenger* took off with a female astronaut on board. Sally Ride became the first American woman in space. It was a big story and *News at Ten* wanted a piece from me.

It was the sort of story I knew I excelled at. Plenty of good pictures, with a strong storyline. I put a report together, and for the last 15 seconds I overlaid a song, 'Ride, Sally Ride', which had been written and recorded to commemorate the event. I was pleased with my efforts.

Sadly, London was not. They took my voice off the report and gave it to a London-based reporter to re-edit and script. That was just about the most humiliating thing they could have done. I was mortified, and maybe for the first time began to understand the true import of what was happening. It seemed that I had gone past redemption. I could have gone up on that shuttle myself, become the first journalist in space, and still they would not have been satisfied.

I didn't know what to do, but knew I had to do something. I felt aggrieved. Were my reports really that poor? Was I failing in the job quite as much as my bosses judged I was? The answers didn't matter. They thought that, and that was all that mattered. Still I pondered what to do. But it wasn't long before my mind was made up for me.

One afternoon the phone in our little love nest rang. It was ITN's managing editor in London. 'The editor wants you in his office tomorrow afternoon, 2 o'clock.' 'But I've ... I'm not sure ... The flights ...' 'Two o'clock tomorrow afternoon, in his office,' and he hung up.

I put the phone down, thought for a moment, and turned to Bon. 'I've got to fly to London tonight. David Nicholas wants me in his office at 2 tomorrow afternoon. I think they may be about to sack me.' I braced myself for I knew not quite what. At the very least, I expected dismay from her, at worst frustration, even anger, that I had allowed things to come to this, put my job on the line, our future at risk.

She smiled. 'That's all right,' she said, 'we'll do something else.'

I remember that moment as if it were yesterday. I can hear the managing editor's voice, remember his words and my words to you exactly, my Bonnie, and of course your response. It was a seminal moment in our fledgling relationship. The full import of it didn't immediately sink in, but it didn't take long. What you were saying was that for us to be together was not only more important than my job but the only thing that truly mattered.

I remember returning your smile, and feeling as if a ton weight had been lifted from my shoulders.

* * * *

Memories. So wonderful when shared, so painful when not. Today is 27th April 2009. I am writing these words 26 years to the day since I collected you at Baltimore Washington airport and we began our life together. I have not mentioned this date to you for some years now, my Bonnie.

Tonight I cooked dinner, a pretty motley affair, which relied on the microwave. We sat eating together, not talking much. You said a couple of things. They made sense, but bore no relationship to what was happening. When I said the carrots tasted good, you said of course they did, you had made them specially.

Then a nice bubble bath, except that for some reason you hate it, and those little sobs as I get you ready cut into me like needles again. But once I get you out, into your nightie and into bed, you are happy. You are sleeping peacefully now as I write about our past together.

We flew to London and took our suitcases to my parents' flat in that block in Baker Street. I walked to ITN in time for my 2 o'clock meeting with the editor. I was in a pretty grim mood, made worse by the few familiar faces I saw in the building, including the receptionist, all looking at me as if I had the plague. Word was out. So was I, or at least I was about to be. I thought better of putting my head round the newsroom door. Frankly I just wanted the axe to fall and the sooner I got out of the building, the better.

Reuters, the BBC and now ITN. All flops. Good going, John. Bon's words were, of course, ringing in my ear, in a kind of gentle sound loop. *That's all right, we'll do something else.* It was wonderful to know I had her support, particularly since I had so little right to expect it. But the question remained: what else could I do apart from journalism? In a word, nothing. I had always wanted to be a professional musician. I wasn't bad on the trombone, but turn professional? I hadn't touched it for 15 years or more. I could busk in a tube station. The thought brought a wry grin to my face.

Even the editor's secretary wouldn't look me in the eye. 'You can go in,' she said, as she tidied some papers on her desk. David Nicholas was sitting behind his desk, a look of thunder on his face. I sat in the single hard chair facing him. He kept his voice low, his natural authority enhanced by the dramatic quality of his Welsh accent.

'I don't know what's happened to you,' he said, 'but you have let me down, me and ITN. You are a disgrace. I gave you the top job because I believed in you, and you have blown it, quite simply blown it. Your reports have been appalling. The Sally Ride piece – you put music on it, for god's sake. What on earth were you thinking about? This is a news organisation, *News at Ten* is the country's premier news bulletin, it's not light entertainment.'

I said nothing. There was nothing to say. I had messed up. But I knew I had Bonnie to go home to. *That's all right, we'll do something else.* He spoke some more. I honestly can't remember what he said. My mind went onto a kind of autopilot, prepared to kick back in when he delivered the *coup de grâce*.

'Right, this is what I have decided. I am bringing you back to London at the end of the year. You will go back on the reporters' desk at the most junior level. It's up to you to work your way back up again.'

I didn't take in the words at first, but ran them rapidly through my mind again. *Back at the end of the year, back on the reporters' desk.* I was dumbfounded, so much so that I actually said, 'Aren't you going to sack me?' The faintest smile played on the corners of his lips, but swiftly disappeared. 'There are those who think I should. Very senior people. But no, I am not going to sack you. You were a good reporter before you went to Washington. That's why I gave you the job. I don't think that has changed. Something has gone badly wrong. I know about your marriage breaking up, and that can't have helped, but that's not why I am keeping you on. I am doing it because I believe you have it in you to put this behind you, and I am giving you the chance to prove me right.'

I thanked him and left.

* * * *

A few years ago, shortly after I had retired from ITN, I received a letter from David Nicholas asking if I would come to south London to give a talk to young people from deprived backgrounds, at an event organised by the charity of which he was President. 'Just tell me where and when, and I'll be there,' I replied.

More recently, in fact only a couple of weeks after I went public about Bonnie's condition, he phoned me. He wanted to tell me how sorry he and his wife were to hear the news, what a lovely person Bonnie was, and how obviously happy we always were. I asked him how he was. 'Pretty good for someone who'll be 80 next birthday,' he replied.

* * * *

In June 1982, Israeli forces had invaded southern Lebanon, then in the autumn there occurred the infamous massacre in the Sabra and Shatila refugee camps, and a year later, in one of the bloodiest phases of the war, more than 10,000 civilians were killed.

Where was I, ace war correspondent, veteran of the Iran Islamic revolution and the Soviet invasion of Afghanistan, in the summer of 1983 as the Middle East burned? In Newport, Rhode Island, covering the America's Cup – and very exciting it was. America was at risk of losing this most prestigious of all sailing trophies for the first time in over a hundred years. A British team was competing, financed by the entrepreneur Peter de Savary, along with teams from other nations, but everybody knew that the team to beat was the Australians. The rumour was that they had a secret revolutionary keel, kept literally under wraps. Every time the yacht was lifted from the water, protective screens went up first.

It was, for a reporter, a peach of a story. It had everything – drama, excitement, rivalry. I got close to the British team, so had plenty of material with which to provide reports for *News at Ten*. I interviewed Alan Bond, the multi-millionaire backer of the Australian team (later to go bankrupt and serve a prison sentence for fraud). I was in exactly the right place at the right time when the American skipper paid an evening visit to the Australian team the night before the final race, having already begun to drown his sorrows at the certainty of defeat the following day. And I was there, with my camera crew, when the Australians finally lifted their yacht from the water with no protective screens, revealing the worst-kept secret in sport, a winged keel.

And would you believe it, my pieces were running – as I had transmitted them by satellite to London – on *News at Ten*. No complimentary messages yet, but it was a start.

Bonnie was with me in Newport, which more than made up for the fact that the only place in the world I really wanted to be was southern Lebanon. I know that sounds a bit bizarre, but from the day I became a reporter all I ever wanted was to be on the biggest story in the world every day. Impossible, of course, but it's what every general news reporter wants. The America's Cup may have been a peach of a story, but I would much rather have been in the infinitely more dangerous Middle East, covering something that would have an impact on the history of the region. The realisation of that brought home to me just how close I had come to scuppering the job I still adored. I was a reporter at heart, it was a reporter I wanted to remain, and thanks to the editor's continuing faith in me, albeit drastically diluted, I still had a chance.

None of these intense thoughts prevented Bonnie and me from enjoying the large jacuzzi bath in the small apartment we were staying in, and locally caught lobster for dinner.

It had to end, of course, and I worked in the Washington bureau with a team who knew I was a lame duck correspondent. The remaining months were painful. There were no more big stories on which I could demonstrate my new-found commitment, and I found myself longing for the end of the year.

It was just as well things were quiet. Bonnie and I were like talking machines. Now that we were together, finally and fully, we just wanted to learn as much about each other as we could. We talked and talked, as we had before, but this time with the warm comfortable feeling that we were together. This wasn't snatched time into which we needed to pack as much as we could. She told me more about her family, her brothers. She said she would love me to meet her family. I'd love her dad, she said. He had mellowed a lot now, but used to be a bit of a tyrant. She described a Sunday lunch when they were all children, and her youngest brother Jon had disagreed with something their dad had said. He exploded. 'Don't you ever question anything I say again!' I told Bonnie that my dad had taught my brothers and me to question everything. She loved that.

She filled me in on her background. She had done well in high school, so well that she was invited to apply for entry into one of America's most prestigious universities, Cornell. She got in, but not in the subject of her first choice. There we found common ground. She had wanted to study the arts, particularly literature, but her dad had thought human ecology was more useful. I had wanted to study modern languages, but the only vacancy was in the social science faculty. We laughed at shared joys and frustrations.

She told me that when she had first come to the UK to marry and settle, she had got a job with the Flour Advisory Bureau on the strength of her Cornell degree. She travelled the UK, lecturing at Women's Institutes on how to make bread. She told me it was part of the rules that she always had to wear a little hat and a two-piece suit. Sixties Britain. God, how we laughed.

That also cleared up a slight mystery. Her American accent had all but disappeared, just small traces remaining in the occasional elongated vowels. Bonnie explained that the Flour Advisory Bureau had told her that in some areas the ladies might find her accent difficult to understand. If she could anglicise it, that would be much appreciated. So she had consciously adopted a more English speaking voice. Ironically, when she went home, her family accused her of snobbishness because she had an English accent.

One evening we went to an all-Beethoven concert at the Kennedy Center. Later I said to her, 'Do you know, one day I would really like to write the story of Beethoven's life.' 'Do it,' she said. 'I think it's a wonderful idea.' I shook my head in disbelief. I still wasn't used to the utter luxury of being with a woman who would support me in whatever I wanted to do, without qualification. It took my breath away.

We returned to London from Washington at the end of 1983. My wife and children would be moving back into the house in Henley, so Bonnie and I had nowhere to live. Don't worry, said my mum, I will fix it, and fix it she did. I couldn't have got a mortgage on a house, having no money whatsoever for a down payment, but I was able to rent a flat because I had a salary from ITN. Mum secured a small flat for us on the top floor of that large mansion block directly over Baker Street tube station, the same block of flats where I spent the first 10 years of my life. Ah yes, the very same block where I had surreptitiously turned up two-and-a-half years before to pay the clandestine visit to my parents.

This is hard to believe, and even harder to write. The intimacy has gone, and it is slowly killing me. There, I have said it.

❋ ❋ ❋ ❋

The task ahead of me was not just daunting, it was well-nigh impossible. Back in London I was *persona non grata*, a leper, unclean. No one would make eye contact, let alone speak to me. I sat at the reporters' desk, my head buried in a newspaper. Less than three years before, I had been not just a popular and gregarious reporter, but lauded by my peers for having secured the impossible, the Washington job. I was the toast of the news-room. My parting gift was a reference to the fact that on my final day in the office before leaving for the States, I had been bought one drink too many by my colleagues – a t-shirt which said 'John Suchet, Newsh at Ten'.

A couple of weeks or so after my return, there was a leaving dinner for a senior ITN executive. I arrived, sat down, and realised fairly quickly that the seats on either side of me were being left empty. No one would sit next to me. Finally a fellow reporter sat beside me, but only because she was a late arrival and there were no other places, and she didn't exchange two words with me throughout the meal. Much later I learned that in the days following she had raised many a smile by saying her career was cursed, she had sat next to John Suchet.

Shortly after this I was summoned by the managing editor – he who had phoned me ordering me back to London to face the editor – to tie up administrative loose ends from my inglorious tenure in Washington. By now the treatment I was receiving was beginning to stir a certain amount of anger in me. Yes, I had failed, yes, I expected no hero's return, but this was all going a bit far.

I sat opposite the managing editor, listening stony-faced as he went through a checklist of issues to do with the house which ITN rented in Washington. Moya and the boys were still over there, and arrangements had to be made to bring them back. The managing editor was a man I had known for more than 10 years, yet the way he was speaking to me, his tone of voice, was that of a headmaster addressing an errant school-boy. Finally I decided to make a stand. I didn't lose my temper, but I came out with a sentence I had prepared, carefully honed, and rehearsed

fast as they could in the opposite direction. I cannot pretend I was totally at ease, but a blast of Beethoven's *Eroica* into my ears from my battered old Walkman gave me the courage I needed and fired me up. A war zone. A big story. At last, at last.

From the moment I set foot on Lebanese soil, it was as if the civil war stopped. It seemed I had brought peace to the region. I managed to get just a single report on *News at Ten* in two weeks, before coming home. Hardly my fault that I had not been given the chance to prove myself, but galling nonetheless.

It wasn't long before I was back in the Middle East. The war between Iran and Iraq was at its height, putting at risk the safe passage of oil down the Gulf, out into the Arabian Sea, and on to the Western world. At the southern end of the Gulf lay the narrow Strait of Hormuz. It was vital that this stretch of water be kept open, and that task fell to Oman. It just so happened the Sultan of Oman was a graduate of Sandhurst, a great Anglophile, and more than happy to have British forces on site to patrol the waters.

ITN dispatched me to cover this British effort for *News at Ten*. I didn't know why it seemed as if I was slowly being brought out of the wilderness, what with Beirut and now this, and I didn't stop to ask. Simple, I hear you say. They were giving you another chance, another opportunity to prove yourself. Television news should work like that, but usually doesn't. Much more likely that the reporter, or reporters, they wanted to send were unavailable for some reason, and yours truly was not.

Whatever the reason, I hooked up with a camera crew and went. I was back in my element: a strong picture story unfolding before me, with British forces naturally keen to get as much favourable coverage as they could, therefore being highly co-operative. I got several reports onto *News at Ten*, and was told on my return they were highly thought of.

More. On 14th June 1985 a TWA passenger plane was hijacked en route from Athens to Rome. With a primed grenade held to his head, the captain defied Beirut control tower and landed. Over the next three days, the plane made four flights between Beirut and Algiers. It wasn't long before they began to carry out their threat to kill passengers. I was sent to cover the Algiers end. There I got close to a senior TWA executive, who, when the drama appeared to be approaching its end, flew my camera crew and me in his executive jet to Athens, allowing us to satellite exclusive coverage to London. More praise.

And then, roll of drums, fanfare, on 7th July 1985 Boris Becker became the youngest-ever player to win the Wimbledon men's title. 'He's flying back to Monte Carlo tomorrow. It's where he trains. Get on the plane with him,' the foreign editor said to me. She didn't need to say it twice, I can tell you.

Despite a thousand media scrumming, pushing, shoving, bribing, to get on that plane, I made it with my camera crew. In Monte Carlo his manager made it clear that there were to be no interviews. I hung around, and got good pictures of Boris, an interview with his manager, and plenty of colour. I satellited my report for *News at Ten*. The foreign news editor made a point of telling me my piece was well received, I had made the story mine, and so I would be sent in a fortnight's time to Becker's home town of Leimen, near Heidelberg, to cover his triumphant return. I duly went, covered the civic reception, filmed young boys on the tennis courts hoping one day to emulate their hero. Becker himself walked out onto the balcony of the town hall, to cheers from the throng below. Again my report was lauded.

Wonder of wonders, people in the newsroom were beginning to talk to me again. I was being treated almost normally. The foreign editor, who had chanced her arm by dispatching me to the Middle East, and to cover Becker, even took me aside to say things were going well for me.

But the rehabilitation was not yet quite as complete as I thought.

* * * *

In London we live in a long narrow apartment, with a corridor that runs the length of it, rooms off to the side. Bon walks up and down this corridor, up and down, day after day. Unless I sit in front of the telly, of course, in which case she comes and sits with me. But if I am at the computer, as I am now, up and down, up and down.

A strange development. Uncanny as it may sound, but if I need to go into the bedroom, to hang something up, say, she is there ahead of me, just a few paces ahead of exactly where I want to be. If I need to go into the kitchen, there she is, just a few paces ahead of exactly where I want to be. Whatever room I am heading for, there she is, exactly a few paces ahead of me.

It made me smile to begin with, now it just makes me cross. This morning was pressured. I needed to wash loads of laundry – her clothes, my clothes, towels, bathroom mat, etc. I was under pressure. I needed to get it done, because I also needed to do some food shopping. Up and down, up and down, always just a few paces ahead of exactly where I needed to be.

I brought some dry T-shirts into the bedroom to hang up, needed to get to the narrow gap between the bed and the cupboards, and yes, bingo, there she was, exactly two paces ahead of me in the narrow gap. I lost it. I walked aggressively on, knocking her out of the way. Yes, you are gasping with horror. So am I, at writing it. But I did it. I had had enough; end of tether time. She cried out and staggered. I opened the cupboard door and hung up the shirts. I pushed past her again. She collapsed on the bed, horror on her face.

I walked back down the corridor, cursing myself out loud. *Why, John, why? Why did you do that? Why?*

She forgot pretty quickly, which is a hallmark of this insidious disease. I too calmed down. We had lunch, and in the afternoon watched snooker on the box. She hasn't the slightest idea of what is happening on the green baize, but as long as I am happy watching, she is happy too.

✳ ✳ ✳ ✳

At the end of 1985, President Ferdinand Marcos of the Philippines called a snap presidential election for March 1986. I'll rephrase that. A nasty corrupt little dictator, kept in power by American backing, called a presidential election in the Philippines that he knew he could rig. To make sure that there would be no surprises, he had taken the sensible precaution of having the opposition leader assassinated. As you do. Interesting story, but interesting enough for the world's media to decide to cover it? No.

But guess what happened then? The assassinated politician's widow announced she would run in her husband's place. Slightly more interesting, but still not quite up there. The Philippines were a long way away, nothing that happened there would have any impact on Britain. However, in the weeks that followed it became clear that the widow's campaign was not some folly, but was attracting growing support, both nationally and internationally. It was becoming front-page news in the British papers.

You didn't need to be an ace journalist to realise this was a good story. But from ITN's point of view it was marginal. A long way away, expensive to cover, when we could easily take in video coverage from local television and the agencies, and voice it in London. I had always adopted a policy of not putting myself forward for a story. I didn't hang around the home and foreign desks, pleading to be sent away. If they want me, let them come to me – a policy that had certainly not helped my cause in the months following my return from Washington.

Since things had been going rather better for me of late, maybe now was the time to be just a little more assertive. I did it on the spur of the moment. In the corridor between the newsroom and the toilets I happened to pass the senior foreign editor – she who had taken me aside to compliment me. 'Er,' I said, trying not to sound too hesitant, 'the, er, Philippines, good story, I was just wondering, if, er, I don't know if you are going to send, but, er, if you did, I would certainly like to, er …'

She cut me short. 'We are not sending. Anyway even if we did, we wouldn't send you.'

If she had punched me in the solar plexus, it would have caused less pain. Damn damn damn, why did I ever ask? I walked back into the newsroom, jaw set, pretending the encounter had never happened.

In television news, things happen more often by accident than by design. The same foreign editor, a few days later, said to me, 'Hope you've been following the Philippines story. We want you to go in a couple of days.' What had made her change her mind? Was the reporter she had in mind unavailable? I soon put all speculation out of my mind. I was going, that was all that mattered.

It truly was an extraordinary story. Corazon Aquino, in her own words a 'plain housewife', was having an impact not just in her own country but around the world. She was in every newspaper, on every television bulletin, as first hundreds, then thousands, then millions of Filipinos poured out onto the streets of Manila, all dressed in yellow – the colour of her party – and all holding up the thumb and forefinger of their right hand, making an L: *Laban*, or Freedom.

Marcos did what dictators do. He ordered the tanks onto the streets to open fire. But the world's television cameras were everywhere. The army dared not. This was to be repeated with much more global impact less than four years later in Berlin and across central Europe, then in Moscow itself. People revolt against dictatorship? No problem, send in the tanks and open fire. But you can't do that when there are cameras present. Still no problem. Censor the coverage, control it. But with satellite technology you can't. The dictatorships of the world were learning a brutal lesson, which would bring their tyrannies to an end. Only in one country could some sort of control be exerted. Thousands died in Tiananmen Square in Beijing when the tanks opened fire. The Chinese put an instant lid on it, but even they could not stop news of the massacre leaking out. The world was changing, and my profession was at the forefront of it. It makes me proud today to think that television news played a part in the downfall of Communism.

And in the downfall of dictator Marcos. He won the election of course, with 99.9999999% of the vote. But Cory (the name by which the world had come to know her) was not giving up. On the same day, in two different parts of Manila, Cory and Marcos were both sworn in as President. For 24 hours, the Philippines had two presidents. But then the Americans told Marcos he was finished, and flew him and his flamboyant wife Imelda out of Manila by helicopter. As the rotor blades whirred overhead, the people stormed the palace and uncovered riches beyond their dreams, not to mention Imelda's 2000 pairs of shoes.

(I can personally vouchsafe for Imelda's ownership of one of the biggest diamond rings I have ever seen. Covering an election rally, we were filming the appalling president and his wife on a small stage that had been erected in a town square. At the end of his speech, they advanced to the front of the stage to extend their hands down to the crowd. I saw Imelda deftly remove the ring from her finger and slip it into her pocket before extending her hands.)

Night after night, I was hitting *News at Ten* with lengthy reports. The world watched the Philippines, fascinated and fixated. Praise was coming back to me from London day after day. I was truly back in my element, doing what I did best. The day after Marcos flew into exile, the city erupted with joy. That, for a journalist, was easy to cover. But what do you do the day after the day the city erupts? You can hardly film it erupting again. Well, that's what the BBC reporter did, but it is not what I did.

I got the one and only scoop of my career. I secured a one-to-one interview with President Corazon Aquino. It led *News at Ten*. How did I achieve this stunning result? By hard work, graft, working the telephones, milking my contacts, journalistic instinct? No. By pure good luck. The right cameraman, the right place, the right time, and a lot of luck. Later, back in London, I was telling a senior colleague just how lucky I had been, and he said, 'Funny how the harder you work, the luckier you get.' I accepted the compliment graciously, but really you don't know just how lucky I had got. Nor am I going to tell you. I shall just allow you to bask in my total rehabilitation as an ITN reporter.

When finally the story was over, the Philippines had its new housewife president, and I arrived home. I opened the front door of the flat and Bonnie was there, waiting for me. She had a huge smile on her face. I expected some sort of questioning, the sort any wife might want to ask of a husband who had just spent several weeks in one of the more exotic countries in the world, where all sorts of sensual delights were readily available. Did she interrogate me? No. She said nothing, took my hand, and led me straight into the bedroom.

I was awarded the Royal Television Society's Journalist of the Year accolade for my Philippines coverage. The citation talked of my 'ability to bring clarity to confused situations'. I mention that for two reasons. My grandfather, the press photographer, gave me a birthday card when I was 10, showing a boy playing a trumpet. Inside it said, 'Blow your own trumpet, because if you don't nobody is going to blow it for you.'

The second reason is just slightly more relevant. Had it not been for Bonnie, her wise words, her encouragement, her belief, her support, her *everything*, not only would there have been no RTS gong, there would have been no career. Left to make my own decision, I would have blown my career clean out of the water (again).

Chapter 4

After we moved to London, just before Christmas 1983, I lost no time in introducing Bonnie to Regent's Park, which Mum had always referred to as our 'back garden' when we were growing up. I walked paths with her I had walked as a kid. I took her to the top of the slope on the other side of the lake. This was where I sat on my tricycle as a toddler, put my arms up so Mum could take off my pullover, lost control of the pedals, sped down the slope, coming off at the bottom by the bridge and skidding along the tarmac. I still have the scar on the back of my left thumb. We laughed and joked and chatted, arms around each other, hugged and kissed. We were teenagers in love.

We bought two gold rings, his and hers, and had them engraved with our initials, J and B. We wear them to this day. Our flat was small, but Bon made it cosy. Our dining table was a small white kitchen table with a flap at each end. Mum and Dad came up for dinner and we squeezed round the little table. God, how happy they were. Not only was their son back in the family, but he was so self-evidently happy. Can a parent want more? Mum and Bon chatted away easily, exchanging female stories and gossip. Dad at one stage caught my eye, emitted a tiny smile and nodded. It was his way of giving a professional judgment, of saying yes, this one is a keeper.

We went to John Lewis and bought a double bed, bedclothes and curtains. Two beanbags served as easy chairs. I bought a cheap and cheerful self-assembly dressing table for Bon, and we laughed together at the mess I made of putting it together. Bon had not worked since a brief spell as an infant teacher following the Flour Council, but now she got a job as a temp and together we could just about afford the rent. We had no intention of staying long. Bon said she didn't want to live in a flat in central London, and was longing for us to get a small house and garden somewhere. I loved living in a flat – albeit small – in the centre of town, but I would have gone to the Highlands of Scotland if she had asked me to.

We stayed in that flat for just under a year, and it was during that time that I served my penance at ITN. It was to that flat I came home with the tears pricking the backs of my eyes, determined to resign. It was during that period that I came to terms with my failure in Washington, that I put my job in perspective, that I came to realise where happiness and fulfillment really lay. And so, as I curbed my ambition and cared rather less about my job, I got better at it.

I retired from ITN at the end of March 2004, to coincide with my big birthday which did not begin with five. I approached that birthday with dread, but Bon, having got there first, helped me through. She was also an integral part of the retirement parties, official and unofficial. After all, had it not been for her, I would have handed in my resignation in a fit of pique many years before. As it was, I stayed at ITN for almost 32 years.

Now, I said to her, we could enter retirement together, do all the things we had planned, go to all the places we had talked about. We could travel Europe, even the world, going to Wagner operas. She smiled weakly.

It was some time in the months following my retirement that a couple of rather odd things happened. I was introducing a Beethoven concert in a large modern concert hall in Milton Keynes. Bonnie was backstage with me in my dressing room. About half an hour before it was due to begin, I walked her out of the dressing room, down a corridor, and pointed to the door she should go through that would lead her into the auditorium, where a seat was reserved for her. I don't know why, some instinct made me watch her as she went. She walked down the corridor and reached the door. She stopped in front of it and hesitated. She reached for the handle, but brought her arm back again. She stood still for a moment, head bowed as if concentrating. Then she looked back round, and her face lit up when she saw me. I hurried towards her. 'Darling, are you alright? What's the matter?' 'I got confused, that's all, I couldn't remember …'

And the second odd thing was that she got lost at Stansted airport that day when we were flying out to France.

✳ ✳ ✳ ✳

Towards the end of 1984, my mother told me she had heard that a much larger flat had become available one floor below. 'Why don't you and Bonnie look at it?' she asked. I said we would, but we also intended starting to look for a small house soon.

As if it were yesterday, I can remember exactly what Bon said and did as we walked round the large empty flat. Doors everywhere, room after room, and something we had none of in the small flat – cupboards. 'Cupboards! At last!' she said. 'Somewhere to put our coats!' We walked the long corridor, marvelling at how many rooms there were. At the far end, the kitchen. We walked in. Bon let out a little yelp and performed a pirouette, arms outstretched. 'It's huge! It's wonderful! We can eat in the kitchen! And look, more cupboards!'

The flat was elegant, with spacious rooms and molded ceilings. Classic 1920s. We walked into the large light bedroom. The ceiling had elaborate molding, in three rectangles, one directly above where the bed would go. Bon looked up at it and said, 'I expect I will spend a lot of time looking up at that.' I laughed out loud at the outrageousness of the remark, basking in a warm glow of expectation.

Oh please let's live here, she implored me. The rent was higher, but by now I knew that at the very worst I was safe in my job, at the best – who could tell, maybe promotion soon? I applied to the landlord and was successful. We moved into the flat at the end of 1984, and I am sitting in it writing this now, almost 25 years later.

I had come home. Not only was I once again living in the same block of flats my brother David and I had grown up in, to be joined later by younger brother Peter, but our new flat was two doors away on the same floor as the flat we had lived in as children. I am at heart a city boy. I loved being back in the centre of London, the noise and bustle, buses and tubes, cafés and shops. Best of all, I could walk to work in 15 minutes, which meant being back with my Bonnie minutes after leaving the office.

Having said that she wanted to move to a little house with a garden in the suburbs, Bonnie soon found that she no longer heard the traffic in the busy road below, and that she didn't miss having a garden quite as much as she thought she would. As I write this, we have been living in Chiltern Court for nearly 25 years.

Small wonder, really, that my job started to go rather well. A close colleague, the reporter and newscaster Carol Barnes, who was to die so tragically young, said to me about this time, 'Do you know, before you went to Washington you were a complete bastard. You argued with everyone. Now you're actually quite nice.'

In the autumn of 2004, my concerns about Bonnie were mounting. An odd remark here or there, something forgotten that should have been remembered, confusion about entries in the kitchen diary – the sort of things you put down to the ageing process, something that happens to us all. But after what had happened at the airport, I couldn't help worrying.

To begin with I joked with Bonnie: 'You've got Alzheimer's, that's what you've got.' It's not really that tasteless – more gallows humour between two people who love each other very much, maybe an attempt to ward off the evil spirits.

But she must have caught the concern in my voice. In the spring of 2005, we were invited to the annual Arnold Bennett commemoration dinner up in his birthplace in the Potteries. I was to give a little speech, then propose a toast to the immortal memory. It was nice to do something so completely different. I am not an Arnold Bennett expert, but I do have something in common with the great under-rated English novelist. I happen to live in the same block of flats in London where he spent his final years and where he died.

We were guests of the chairman of the Arnold Bennett Society and his wife. Both utterly charming. But the chairman saddened when he told us his wife had Alzheimer's. 'You can't tell just talking to her,' he said. 'In fact, you probably haven't noticed anything at all. But she has it.'

On the way home after the event, I remarked on how sad it was to hear the chairman's wife had Alzheimer's. 'That's what you think I have,' Bon said to me, smiling. I was caught totally by surprise. 'What? Of course I don't.' 'Yes you do,' she said, still smiling, 'and just in case you're in any doubt, I don't have it.'

Bon and I wanted to get married as soon as possible, but we both had to get divorced first. Her husband was more sad than angry, realised it was something he couldn't fight, and agreed to a simple and speedy divorce. Bon's children, Alec the eldest and Hereward (universally known as H), both teenagers, were bewildered and sad, but we did all we could to welcome them to the flat and make them feel at home. There was no easy way to explain why we had to do what we had done, but we assured them of constant love and attention.

My wife was more angry than sad, and the divorce was a long drawn-out process. One remark sticks in my mind. At a session with my solicitor, he said 'Normally a divorce case will fill a fairly thick file, if it's a complicated one it might fill a drawer.' He then pointed to an entire row of filing cabinets and said, 'Yours has filled all of them, and we're not through yet.' From work I would phone Bon each morning and say, 'Any bad post today?' There was barely a day, certainly not a week, without a legal letter several pages long that needed a response.

The case went to the High Court in the summer of 1984. I remember it in the way you remember a bad dream. A solicitor who was eating up practically every spare penny ITN was paying me, and now a barrister. His fees, well, they really were a sick joke. I tried to telephone him once. His clerk expostulated down the phone, 'Speak to him? Speak to him, sir? You want to speak to him? Utterly absurd, absolutely out of the question. You must speak to your solicitor. Only he is allowed to speak to counsel. You must be totally mad, an idiot, sir, d'you hear me?' All right, I made the last bit up, but the rest is true, and honestly I think if I had telephoned Buckingham Palace and asked to speak to the Queen, I would have elicited a less dismissive response.

The case took a whole day in the High Court – that over-ornate building at the top of the Strand, which I had attended so many times as a reporter. We went before Mr Justice Somebody-or-Other in the morning, then the two competing barristers went into a huddle, then before him again. In the afternoon I remember seeing the two barristers strolling together in the vast hall of the building, while I sat with my solicitor on a stone step. My about-to-be ex-wife was in an alcove with her solicitor. The barristers were chatting together, occasionally gesturing, occasionally smiling. I imagine the conversation went something like this. 'I say, old chap, huntin' this weekend?' 'Actually yes, old boy, and you?' 'Fishin' meself, and a bit of shootin'.' 'What about this case? Simple enough, but let's keep talkin', eh? Make it last a few more hours, should do wonders for the fees, what?' 'He-he, totally, I should co-co, me ol' sport.' Something like that, anyway.

It all ended at around 8pm, with me surrendering all I had. A huge monthly payment amounting to half my net salary – yes, half my *net* salary – for the children, plus the house in its entirety, and everything in it. Barristers had gone, probably off to have a glass of bubbly together. Even my solicitor had vanished. The vast cavernous space was empty.

But it was over, at last. Well, sort of. There were court orders, which resulted in my not seeing the children for the best part of three years. Nor were my parents allowed to see their first grandchildren, which distressed them. *Déjà vu* again? Most certainly. Didn't see my parents for those long years, now it was my children I wasn't seeing. It was a traumatic time for me, but I had my Bonnie's arms to fall into whenever I needed comforting. In my own melodramatic way I wondered if I would ever see my boys again, let alone be able to repair in some measure the damage. It took a while, but things did work out in the end. Thank God. I know that what Bonnie and I did hurt our children, all five of them, but today relationships all round are normal, with another grandchild due any day. I really do have a lot to be thankful for.

In March 2005 we went up to see Bon's son H and his young family in the fine old house he and his wife had bought in a village in Lincolnshire. H gave us a guided tour. 'Still a lot of work to do,' he said, 'and one of the most important things is to put in a downstairs toilet.'

Half an hour or so later, Bonnie said she needed to spend a penny. 'Up the stairs,' said H, 'turn left at the top, and it's the door facing you.' 'Don't worry,' said Bon, 'I'll use the downstairs one.'

A little later Bon was confused about where she had put her handbag. I paid no attention, but I caught the look of consternation on H's face. Shortly before we left to come home, H took me to one side. 'I am worried about Mum,' he said, 'she seems very confused.' He mentioned the toilet confusion, and what had happened with her handbag. 'I think you need to see someone. A doctor.'

His words shouldn't have hit me as hard as they did. I saw in an instant that clue after clue that something was happening had presented themselves, but I was simply batting them away. What he said confirmed what my subconscious was telling me, but what I was, I suppose, refusing to confront.

I booked an appointment with our GP.

And so came my first encounter with the cognitive and memory test. All medics acknowledge that it is pretty unscientific, but it at least gives an indication of what may be going on with the brain.

It's nothing more than a series of questions, and it can vary from test to test, doctor to doctor. But generally speaking, it goes something like this: 'What city are we in? ... What sort of building is this? ... Who is the Prime Minister? ... What day is it today? ... I am now going to give you three words to remember, and I will ask you what the words are at the end of the test – tree, house, ball ... Spell 'world' backwards ... Here's a number, 92, take 7 away, take 7 away, take 7 away, take 7 away, until you can't take 7 away any more ... Now what does this picture show? ... Can you draw these shapes? ... And so on, and so on, until finally, 'What were the three words I asked you to remember?'

Bon sat opposite our GP and performed stunningly. She was a bit hesitant in places, but always came up with the answer. She made only one mistake. She spelled 'world' backwards incorrectly. At the end the GP said she really couldn't take it any further, since there was no obvious sign of cognitive impairment. But she said I should keep an eye on things and contact her again if anything further happened.

Bonnie, by the way, sat happily bemused through the whole thing, not once asking what it was all about.

Some months passed, then came Atlanta and our world changed forever.

* * * *

Bonnie and I were married on 29th June 1985. In contrast to both our first marriages, this was a small private affair. Bonnie wore a salmon-pink chiffony two-piece, all pleats and gentle folds, which swayed alluringly as she moved. I wore a rather stylish (though I say it myself) white jacket I had bought in Paris covering the 40th anniversary of the D-Day landings the year before. The venue was Marylebone Register Office in central London, a short walk from our flat. Mum and Dad were there, close family and just a very few close friends, no more than a dozen in all. For the ceremony we had agreed we would use the gold rings with our initials on them. At the appropriate moment I put hers onto the third finger of her left hand, because that was where she wore it. No, said the Registrar gently, the fourth finger. There was stifled laughter.

Some months later we went to the US to see Bon's family. Her father, an elder of the church, wanted us to receive a religious blessing. Bon, knowing my views on religion, asked me tentatively if I would mind. Of course not, I said. I would have crawled to the altar on broken glass if she had asked me. It'll just be a blessing, I promise, she said. In the event, her Dad had laid on a full-blown wedding ceremony. Not a big affair, just the family, but the whole ritual, beginning with a session with the minister. Bon looked at me in panic. Why should I have minded? I didn't, in the least. If it made her dad happy, that was fine by me. My only concern came when we knelt at the altar. I hoped to hell I hadn't worn my shoes with the soles that needed repair. Bon wore those cream combs and looked utterly stunning.

On 25th October 2005 I received a phone call that blew me off my feet. It was from an old colleague at ITN by the name of Chris Shaw, previously a senior *News at Ten* programme editor, now head of news at Channel Five television. He told me the presenter of *Five News* Kirsty Young (also a former colleague at ITN) was going on maternity leave in the New Year, and he wondered if I fancied doing a little bit of newscasting, just a couple of months or so. I would like to say I was shocked speechless, but in fact I burst out laughing.

'Absolutely not,' I said, 'I haven't had an earpiece in my ear for nearly two years. I wouldn't risk it.' 'Don't be daft,' he said, 'it's like riding a bike. You'll pick it up again as if you've never been away.' I said no again, but agreed to have lunch with him.

A former colleague, plus the *Five News* editor, the three of us talking television news, old stories, much laughter, familiar names. I was back in my element, my world. It was 18 months since I had left ITN, since I had in effect retired from newscasting. Just three months before, on 7th July, the London bombings had happened. I watched the news coverage with an ache in my heart, a pit in my stomach. This was the biggest story in the UK for very many years, and I wasn't involved. I was out of news.

'Do you know what?' I had said to Bonnie. 'I've left it behind. I've moved on. Even if they rang and asked me, I would say no.' Then they rang and asked me.

So, no surprise, I agreed to go back into the studio. Chris said Kirsty was planning to go on leave in late January or early February. 'Let's talk in terms of Easter,' he said, 'late January to Easter, a couple of months. What do you say?'

I ran it past Bonnie. She said if it was what I wanted to do, she would certainly not try to stop me. Then I had an inspiration. 'I know what. Let's go to the States before then and see your family.'

We hadn't seen Bonnie's brothers and their wives for some time, nor had I seen my son Rory in Atlanta for a while, so I planned a rather complicated – but exciting – trip for the dog days at the end of November 2005, the mellow days of autumn gone, but the joy of Christmas not yet in full swing. We would fly to Philadelphia, connect for the flight down to Atlanta, spend three days with Rory, fly back up to Philly, spend three days with the family, then back home.

It got off to a difficult start. Bon had trouble packing, but this was nothing new and I sort of expected it. It was just one of those things. For years, whenever we travelled she found packing – clothes selection – really difficult. It didn't matter, I was used to it. Anyway, by now I knew her clothes and requirements better than she did. I packed for us both. We left good and early for the mid-morning flight from Heathrow. We checked in, went through passport control, and headed to a café to relax for half an hour before our flight was called. Everything had gone smoothly, no unexpected hold-ups despite the increased post 9/11 security, and we were in buoyant and excited mood.

Then Bonnie said she needed to spend a penny. I don't know why I tensed up; after all, there's nothing wrong with wanting to freshen up after a coffee and croissant and before a transatlantic flight. But alarm bells went off in my head. I looked around to locate the toilets and with huge relief saw that they were just 20 metres or so away, down a corridor off to the right from the café. I pointed to them, told her I would stay right here at the table, and off she went.

Five minutes, 10, 15, and that familiar old feeling of tension in the stomach transmuted in a split second into total panic. I prayed we weren't going to have a repeat of what happened at Stansted. It had been some time before, nothing as serious had happened since, and I had practically put it out of my mind. Suddenly it came flooding back. I fixed my eyes on the entrance to the toilet. Women coming and going. Should I ask one to check for me? She must be inside. I surely couldn't have missed her if she had come out already. I had hardly taken my eyes off the entrance. I braced myself to approach a woman to ask for help.

'*May I have your attention please. Would Mr John Suchet please come to the information desk.*'

I sighed to myself, no anger this time, just a wearying sense of *déjà vu*, blended with a feeling of relief that she was at least safe, not collapsed in a toilet cubicle. And there was the beaming smile of recognition when she saw me, just like last time. I had longer to reflect on it in the plane this time. What did it mean? Should I get her checked out again? It was a worry.

✳ ✳ ✳ ✳

We had a belated honeymoon in 1986, nearly a year after our wedding, on the Greek island of Skopelos. I had just returned from the Philippines, so was in need of a break. We became friendly with the young couple, Theo and Eleni, whose small hotel we stayed in. It was their first year in business. We danced Zorba-style with them, laughed and drank with them. Bonnie said to me one night she could see sadness in Theo's eyes. I was taken aback. He seemed a thoroughly cheerful chap, and I told her I was sure she was wrong. Feminine instinct. I still didn't realise just how powerful it was.

In conversation I had mentioned that my father was a gynaecologist and obstetrician, albeit retired. Theo took me aside one evening and told me he and Eleni had tried everything to have a baby, but nothing worked. They had now been told by a specialist that there was nothing else that could be done. Would I mind asking my dad if he thought anything could be tried in London?

Of course I wouldn't. When we got home I had a word with Dad, and he was very pessimistic. If they came to London, it would cost them a lot of money to have IVF treatment, he said, with the odds overwhelmingly stacked against success. He said that if they were determined, they should contact the Cromwell Hospital in Knightsbridge, which was a leader in the field. I took it upon myself to get a brochure from the hospital, which I forwarded to Theo, along with Dad's cautionary advice.

Theo wrote back immediately, saying he was so grateful and that Bonnie and I were dear friends because of what I had done. He said if ever we wanted to return to Skopelos, all we needed to do was book the flights and a room would be waiting. As it turned out, they never did have children, but we nearly took up his offer 21 years later, when we got in touch again through a mutual friend. I considered visiting them in July 2007, but that was one-and-a-half years after Bon's diagnosis, and the dementia was beginning to take hold. I decided against it, not just because I was worried about Bon, but because honestly I didn't think I could have gone back with her to that hotel without cracking up.

❋ ❋ ❋ ❋

November 2005. We landed at Philadelphia airport on time, giving us an easy couple of hours to make our domestic connection down to Atlanta. We were due in Atlanta at 7pm, perfectly in time for a great dinner with Rory. Didn't work out quite that way.

Our connecting flight was delayed indefinitely because of storms. I phoned Rory on my mobile and he said he wasn't surprised – the skies over the city were dark and heavy, flashes of lightning and gusts of wind. I said something irrational about how come we could fly men to the moon but couldn't fly aeroplanes in a storm. I was tired, so was Bonnie. In fact, she looked exhausted.

We sat in the departure lounge for five hours. By the time we got to Atlanta we were drained of any energy. Fatigue was no stranger to Bonnie, but it was not something I often suffered from. If I was now exhausted, I could scarcely imagine how Bonnie must feel. But she didn't complain, not once. I wanted to blame someone, or something, for the fact that we arrived in Atlanta so late, but Bonnie just kept saying how fortunate we were to have got down there at all that night.

Rory fed us late, knocked us out with a bottle of wine, took us down to the guest apartment in his block, and we slept for our country. The next day he took us in to CNN, we met his colleagues, had a leisurely lunch, then returned to our small apartment where Bon had a good rest and I listened to some music. We arranged to meet in his apartment at seven.

Once there, he opened a bottle of red wine. Bon was well rested and on good form. The moment she sat on the sofa, one of his two cats came straight across the room and leapt onto her lap. We laughed and chatted. He had booked a table at a Japanese restaurant just a two-minute walk away.

I took pictures. Bonnie is happy and smiling in them. There is absolutely no hint of what was about to happen.

We polished off the wine, Bon drinking just two small glasses. She reluctantly lifted the cat off her lap, and we walked out into the muggy Atlanta air – not cold, even in late November. We were shown to a window table; Rory sat on one side, Bon and me opposite.

The manageress came straight over to our table, told us she was from Ireland, and said she had grown up watching me read the news on television. It was a strange sort of conversation to be having in a Japanese restaurant in Atlanta.

We ordered wine, I poured, Bon took a sip, and we ordered. The first dishes of raw fish arrived. In-between words and laughter, I began to eat. Suddenly Rory said, 'Dad, look. Bonnie!'

I turned to my left. Bonnie's head had slumped forward, her chin on her chest. 'Darling! Love!' I lifted her chin up and gasped out loud. Her eyes were open and her pupils had rolled up into the top of her head so that I could just see their lower rim below her upper eyelids. Otherwise her eyes were entirely white. She was unconscious, clearly, and I realised immediately it might be very, very serious. 'Get an ambulance!' I said to Rory. He darted out from the table and ran to the reception desk.

I called her name into her ear in a hoarse whisper. I slapped her cheeks, trying to be gentle. 'Darling! Stay awake! Stay awake!' I kept slapping her cheeks, but there was no reaction. Her head dropped back down. I lifted it up again. 'Stay awake, darling! Stay awake!' Some vague remembrance stirred at the back of my head that you should always try to keep someone awake if they have passed out, not let them succumb to sleep. I didn't know if this was one of those occasions. The more likely explanation for my behaviour, looking back on it, is that I wanted some evidence that would show she was still alive.

That came after about two or three minutes. Eyes still open and white, pupils still all but vanished up into her head, suddenly she yawned. She was alive. I let out a huge sigh of relief, but continued slapping her cheeks even more gently, and telling her to stay awake, stay awake.

Then I saw – and I remember it so vividly now nearly four years later – her pupils slowly slide down into their rightful position as if in gently oiled slow motion. Next a small smile slowly spread across her face as she recognised me. 'Darling, darling,' I said, tears welling up in my eyes, 'Are you alright?' 'I think so,' she said in a tiny whisper. 'What happened?'

'You … you fainted, you passed out, but … Thank God you're alright now.'

I was distracted by a small commotion in the aisle next to me. A young man in casual clothes with a totally bald head was crouched down beside me. 'Eh oop, what's all this then?' Yes, the lead paramedic from the fire station just 50 metres down the road was a Yorkshireman from Leeds. He took one look at Bonnie and realised he wasn't dealing with some over-excited individual who had drunk themselves unconscious.

'Y'awright, luv?' he asked. 'Tell ya what, we'll get you to a 'ospital as quick as we can and let 'em tek a good look at yer.'

With his colleague he put up a stretcher on wheels, lifted Bon onto it, and wheeled her out of the restaurant, Rory leading the way and me bringing up the rear.

❋ ❋ ❋ ❋

The paramedics wheeled the stretcher up the ramp into the ambulance and told me I could sit with her. The Leeds lad drove, while his colleague set up a drip to get saline into Bonnie's bloodstream, and took readings of her vital signs. After a few minutes he turned to me and said, 'All looks fine.'

What I remember most vividly is that Bonnie didn't stop smiling and squeezing my hand. The driver must have radioed ahead, because there was an emergency team waiting at the hospital to take over. They wheeled her into a curtained-off area. I thanked my Leeds friend and his colleague and went to join her.

Two nurses fussed around her. Another drip went up, a clip went onto her forefinger, various other wires and paraphernalia were attached, and soon the monitor they were connected to was a moving screen of jagged lines. And still she smiled at me.

The nurses went about their business without saying a word. Then into the next cubicle to check on somebody else. Then back again to monitor those jagged lines. So it continued for the best part of an hour. Finally I decided to say something. 'Er, can you tell me if my wife is alright? Can you tell what happened?' 'The emergency doctor will be around soon. You can speak to him.'

A little bolt of anger shot through me before I remembered these medics were in the process of keeping people alive who might not otherwise be. Their job was to ensure survival until more highly qualified medics could take over. I sent Rory home and settled down for what I was beginning to realise would be a long haul. My anxiety had largely passed. Bonnie was smiling, talking, and apart from looking weak and drained, seemed to be behaving as if nothing had happened. All that medical stuff attached to her was the only graphic reminder of the scene in the restaurant.

The doctor came in two or three hours later, somewhere around midnight. He checked all the vital signs, asked me to describe what had happened, and carried out a swift examination. I was expecting a diagnosis, an answer. I was expecting him to say, 'She's had a such-and-such, or a this-or-that.' For the first time I truly understood what my dad used to say, that patients always want a diagnosis.

But he was totally non-committal, said they would carry out more tests in the morning, and then he was gone. The nurse said they would wheel Bon's bed into a small area, which they could curtain off, and she could sleep till morning. I could go home, the nurse said. Yeah, right, like I would. Bon quickly fell asleep, I stretched out my legs in the chair and so did I.

* * * *

A more senior doctor came to see Bonnie in the morning and went through the whole thing again. At the end he said, 'We need to establish why your wife passed out. So far there is no indication. We'll need to carry out tests. It means staying here all day. Is that alright?' I said of course it was.

To be honest, the day passed in a bit of a blur. I was pretty exhausted, having snatched no more than an hour or two's sleep in the chair. I remember they took blood from Bon, monitored her heart, put her through a series of movement tests, and so on. Everything took longer than expected, not least because the hospital was absolutely huge, and it took 15 minutes or more just to get from one department to another, with a hospital porter pushing Bon in a wheelchair.

By the end of the day, a nurse told us rather apologetically that the main test, the most important one of all, an MRI scan of the brain, would have to wait until the next morning.

Bonnie now had her own room, was clearly on the mend, and I felt I could safely leave her. I went back to the guest apartment and slept deeply. I returned to the hospital bright and early the next morning, and walked with the porter as he wheeled Bonnie what seemed like miles to the MRI scanning department.

It was extraordinary, like walking into a nuclear bunker. Danger signs everywhere, huge imaging machines, everybody wearing spacesuits. A technician who looked ready to walk on the moon wheeled my poor frail little Bonnie into a dark room and told me to keep well away.

Over the next hour there were comings and goings of astronauts, lots of clicking, whirring and buzzing. Finally my Bonnie emerged, looking tired, her hair a mess, but none the worse for wear. We went back up to her room and both fell asleep. I remember thinking as I drifted off, 'I hope we wake up again.'

Some time around mid-afternoon a senior doctor came to see us, holding a clipboard bristling with printed sheets. I could see graphs, arrows, numbers.

'Well,' she said, shaking her head, 'we really are rather mystified. We just don't know why you lost consciousness, ma'am. I have all the test results here. Your blood is fine, your heart is fine, and the MRI scan doesn't show up anything untoward. What I think we can say is that you did not have a heart attack, and you did not have a stroke. Those would be the two most likely things to have caused it.'

There was silence. Where was the diagnosis? I wanted a diagnosis. It seemed I wasn't going to get one. I truly didn't know what to say. But the doctor continued, 'I should say one thing. We didn't carry out a full MRI, just a basic one to establish no obvious stroke. The scan does show a small amount of abnormal white matter in the brain, but that is not consistent with a stroke.'

I pounced on that. 'A small amount of … er … abnormal? There is something abnormal? What does that mean?'

'It's not clear,' she said, 'but it almost certainly has nothing to do with what happened to your wife. It might be due to some underlying cause, maybe a degenerative disease like Alzheimer's.' My gasp was audible. She continued, 'Whatever it is, one thing is certain. What happened to your wife should not have happened. Something went wrong, and you should establish what it was. When you return to London, I suggest you have her thoroughly checked out.'

Bonnie said nothing during any of this. She asked no questions, showed no signs of alarm or even disquiet. She was clearly happy to let me do all the questioning. But that's Bonnie.

The hospital discharged her, with the advice that we shouldn't go up to Philadelphia as planned. Also, the doctor recommended, we should stay three or four more days in Atlanta to allow Bonnie to rest fully and to make sure that there was no repeat of what had happened. We returned to our apartment. I phoned one of her brothers in Haddonfield, New Jersey, and told him the worrying news. He said he would pass it on to the family, had a nice chat on the phone with Bon, and wished her well. Rory secured an extension on the apartment for us, and we settled in for a few days' rest.

We left for London the following Monday. On the British Airways plane, we were assigned two seats right at the back of the plane, just in front of the toilets and a wall, which meant we couldn't recline. I cursed my meanness. Why had I not simply booked us first class, whatever the cost? Bonnie was still exhausted, despite the few days' rest. An overnight flight to London, without being able to recline even a little, would be awful for her. Damn, damn, damn, I thought. If ever I should have not counted the cost, this was the time. I apologised to Bonnie over and over again. She just smiled at me weakly, not uttering a word of complaint.

We took off, dinner was served, and suddenly a stewardess was kneeling by our seats. 'Mr Suchet?' she asked in a quiet voice. 'Yes,' I said. 'Welcome aboard, sir. Some months ago we had the pleasure of flying your brother to Los Angeles, and now it is a pleasure to be flying you and your wife. Would you please both follow me ...'

We followed her up the aisle, into World Traveller Plus, into Business, and still she kept walking. All the way to the front, where a small team of smiling cabin crew waited to welcome us. We were served a wonderful meal, then one of the crew made up a full-length bed for Bonnie. As she prepared to lie down she smiled at me, started to speak, but she was asleep before her head reached the pillow. Thank you, British Airways. Thank you, brother David. Sometimes it really is useful to have a brother who is a famous actor.

Back in London we went to see a neurologist. He said he would carry out a full range of tests on Bonnie, which would require her to be admitted to hospital for five days. It was a few days before Christmas, so he suggested some time in January. He made a couple of phone calls, and we put 9th January 2006 in the diary.

It was the worst scenario imaginable for me. Remember that phone call out of the blue? I had agreed to start at *Five News* on 12th January. Bonnie would be in hospital, and I would be worried sick about her. At the same time I would be in a strange newsroom, with people I didn't know, learning a new computer system, with just a few days' rehearsal in a new studio, presenting a new programme format on live television. To say I felt overwhelmed would be an understatement. I was crushed.

I remember vividly, on the evening of 11th January, standing by the window in Bonnie's hospital room. She lay in bed, exhausted from all the tests. The most important one of all – a full MRI brain scan – was scheduled for the next day. I was due to go live on Channel Five the next day. It was dark outside, with an icy drizzle. In the morning, when Bonnie's head disappeared underneath the scanner – 'Keep still, try to keep absolutely still, push this button if you feel unwell' – I wouldn't be there to comfort her. I would be in a studio, ruining a reputation built on 30 years of live television news broadcasting. I went home that night to an empty flat, feeling utterly disconsolate. How could our lives have suddenly been blown so totally off course?

I got away with it in the television studio. In fact, I continued to get away with it for the next two years, which in the event were perhaps the most rewarding two years of my career, ending with that unexpected and undeserved gong. I found myself schooling a new generation, young journalists who told me they had grown up with me, little expecting to work with me. Gratifying, to put it mildly. But I knew none of that when

I took Bonnie to the National Hospital for Neurology for the final set of tests. These tests were a vastly expanded version of the cognitive test our GP had given her almost a year before.

In the event, she was closeted in a room with a specialist for three hours. She finally emerged and gave me a broad smile of relief. The specialist said to me, gently and quietly, 'It might be a good idea to take certain measures to make things easier. For instance, a diary always open to the right date. Make lists for everything. Keep things in the same place, don't move them around too much. You might want to put a sign on the toilet door. Familiarity. That's the key word.' I don't know why, but I had been kind of hoping the specialist would say everything was fine, and why on earth had I ever thought otherwise? I nodded and thanked her, with a heavy sense of foreboding.

It was a month before we got the results. On 15th February 2006, I walked with Bonnie up the steps of the Lindo Wing of St Mary's Hospital – the steps brother David and I had walked up many times with Dad, who had worked there for 30 years or more, in fact the steps both he and I, and later my younger brother Peter, had been carried down by Mum days after our birth. I felt Dad heavy on my shoulder as I guided Bonnie gently into the consulting room to see the neurologist. With my over-developed sense of the melodramatic, I wondered if the room we were in was the room in which I had been born. It was possible.

We sat opposite him and he came straight to the point. 'Mr and Mrs Suchet, hello again. So nice to see you. Right, I've now had the results of all the tests we did. Mrs Suchet, I am very sorry to have to tell you I believe you have a degenerative brain disease, possibly Alzheimer's.'

We immediately turned to each other. I smiled, put my arm round her, and said, 'It's fine, darling, don't worry, it's fine.' I could scarcely believe it, but she smiled back at me, as if she hadn't understood, but also with the certainty that if I was saying everything was fine, then it really was. 'Oh good,' she said.

The neurologist put the brain scans up on an x-ray window. He pointed to some minute areas, not much more than pinpricks, which were black. 'They should be white,' he said. I heard the word 'hippocampus', then something about 'ischemic' which I didn't understand at all. What really struck me was that he was actually quite hesitant about the diagnosis. Everything he said was peppered with 'maybe', 'might', 'possibly', and so on.

I decided to reduce the conversation to basics. 'I've noticed that if Bonnie goes shopping for food, she'll come back with a dozen yoghurts … She doesn't make lists any more, or if she does they don't make sense.' I was aware that hearing me talk about her like this might upset Bonnie, or at least confuse her. But again she said nothing. When I smiled at her, which I did again and again, she always smiled back.

Expecting the neurologist to be impatient to return to medical terms, I was surprised that he was extremely interested in what I was saying. In fact, he questioned me about it, and asked for more examples. I realised then that he was actually looking for back-up, confirmation of his diagnosis, as if even with all the test results, the MRI scans up on the windows, he was still not sure beyond any doubt.

Finally I said, 'So we know it's Alzheimer's, do we?' 'It's impossible to be absolutely sure,' he said. 'Bonnie has dementia, which is a degenerative disease of the brain. There are over a hundred causes of dementia. We'll call this Alzheimer's, because it is the most common, and we will be treating it in the same way.'

This entire conversation took place without Bonnie saying a word, or reacting in any way. It was really quite odd.

I was calm as we walked down those Lindo Wing steps. I was making a mental note of the things I had to do. Tell the boys, to start with. Arrange to see our GP, make sure I had a prescription for the Aricept the neurologist had prescribed. The irony was not lost on me that as a newscaster I had delivered countless stories on the controversy surrounding the availability of Aricept to people in the early stages of Alzheimer's; now here I was, preparing to get a supply for my Bonnie.

I knew there was a long road ahead, that it would get progressively worse, that our lives would change. I said none of this to Bonnie as we walked to the main road to catch a cab. All I said was, 'He's a nice chap, that brain quack, isn't he?' 'Yes, really nice,' she said.

Back home, and in the days following, I said nothing about the diagnosis, and Bonnie never mentioned it. Did she understand it? Had she taken it in? I honestly had no idea. The likelihood was that she hadn't, otherwise surely she would have said something? To this day, more than four years later, she still has said not a word about it. I most certainly have never asked, and never will.

Chapter 5

David Nicholas, editor-in-chief of ITN, called me into his office some time in the early summer of 1986, post Philippines, post honeymoon. I can't deny a slight tremor, a tiny feeling of apprehension caused by the memory of the last somewhat one-sided conversation I'd had with him in this same room.

His secretary smiled at me this time. I knocked and went in, and couldn't see him at first. He wasn't sitting behind the desk, that single hard chair no longer opposite him. He was in the process of carrying a comfortable armchair across the office to face another one. He gestured to me to sit, put his chair down and sat a couple of feet away from me. His face had a sunny and bright smile on it.

He opened the conversation with an amiable comment, and was soon lauding me for my Philippines coverage, especially that scoop of an interview with Madame President. I calculated instantly that this was not the moment to give him chapter and verse of the outrageous piece of luck that had played into my hands. I decided instead to smile, and bask – albeit modestly – in his praise. But I couldn't help wondering what else he might be about to say. He couldn't have called me in simply to talk of the Philippines. In news terms, that was already ancient history.

Nothing could have prepared me for what he said next. 'I want you to be a newscaster. I am taking you off the road, and I want you to be a full-time newscaster.' He went on to explain that a new television channel, horribly named Superchannel, was launching early the following year, its remit to broadcast the best of the BBC and ITV across Europe. The channel wanted ITN to provide a nightly news specially made for the channel, with an international agenda. 'And I want you to present it.'

I was temporarily lost for words. 'But ... but ...' He smiled, 'I think you will make a good newscaster.' I shook my head. 'But ... I am a reporter. That's what I love. Reporting. I don't want ... I mean, to come inside, into the studio, it's not ...'

He dismissed my half-hearted protests with a wave of the hand. He explained just what an exciting venture this was. Never before had television been broadcast from London across Europe. At least 16, maybe more, countries would fall into the 'footprint' of the satellite. 'You will be seen nightly across Europe,' he said. He told me he had chosen me because I had a clear speaking voice without a strong regional accent, and a friendly and approachable face. I leaned forward to see if I could detect any sign that this was somehow a joke, that he was having a laugh at me. But it appeared he meant it. He mentioned the little bit of part-time newscasting I had already done, and said he thought I had taken to it rather well. I shook my head. My view was different. 'We launch on 2nd February,' he said.

When I finally found my voice, and after a very swift piece of thinking, I said, 'If it doesn't work out, I mean if it turns out I am no good as a newscaster, can I go back to reporting, at the same level I'm at now?' 'Of course,' he said, but there was no conviction in his voice.

In August 1986 I came off the road, after a decade of reporting which had taken me to every country in Western Europe, as well as the Middle East, India and Pakistan, Africa, the Americas, the Far East. I had been arrested and expelled from Iran, Afghanistan and Poland (twice). I had interviewed presidents, prime ministers, Olympic gold medallists, Oscar winners, prisoners on death row, pop stars and fraudsters. I had stayed in some of the world's best hotels, and slept on the street. I had eaten in some of the world's best restaurants, and gone without food. Margaret Thatcher, under intense pressure after the sinking of the Argentine navy cruiser *Belgrano*, answered my aggressive questioning with dignity and courtesy. Supermodel Twiggy, unhappy with a question I put to her, threatened to smash my bleedin' face in. (In a misguided attempt to endear myself to her with a bit of plain Cockney speaking, I suggested to her that her newborn baby daughter had not yet inherited her mother's looks – something that led *my* mum to ask, incredulous, 'Are you really telling me you suggested to a mother her baby was not beautiful?')

I came off the road, fully expecting to be back out reporting again in a matter of weeks. In the event, I remained a full-time newscaster for the next 20 years, until the end of my career with ITN.

* * * *

Some time after we got the diagnosis, I was preparing dinner. Bonnie walked into the kitchen and made a really funny joke about having Alzheimer's. Clever, witty, it took me totally by surprise. I laughed out loud, and she joined in with me. I chuckled all the following day, and at dinner when I reminded her of it we both laughed out loud again.

The next morning I couldn't remember what it was she had said, and I can't remember to this day.

In the weeks and months following the diagnosis, the single biggest fear I had was that I would develop dementia too. Why not? Why should I be immune? The disease is not in Bonnie's family, and it is not in mine – at least as far back as it is possible to know. Deafness was not in Beethoven's family, either. What if I developed it and was no longer able to look after Bonnie?

That was just one of the unknowns. How would the disease progress in Bonnie? I started reading up about it, as you do. *Most sufferers die within 10 years of diagnosis … We are all living longer, therefore more and more of us will develop dementia … How I watched my elderly mother disappear before my eyes …*

Cheery stuff. Really uplifting. I learned one thing, and one thing only. No one knows anything. I mean that. No one knows anything about any of it – not the scientists, not the doctors, not the sufferers, not the carers, nobody.

At a recent wedding, an old friend of the family said that looking at me was like looking at my mum. I had her looks, her characteristics, I spoke in a similar way, and had her smile. Brother David was more like Dad, Peter a nice combination of both. I knew she was right; in fact, I reinforced what she said by telling her I had followed Mum's dad into photo/TV journalism. I've got the Jarché genes, I told her.

But one thing I inherited from Dad, in spades. His cynicism. And so I shall have a little rant, and plead your tolerance (if forgiveness is too much to ask). In his retirement, Dad found a sentence in some article somewhere that really tickled him; tickled him so much, in fact, that he cut it out and sellotaped it to the wall above his desk. It read:

The practice of medicine is harmful to the health.

Remember, this was one of London's best-known and most highly respected gynaecologists and obstetricians, a fellow of the Royal College of Surgeons. When I first saw the quote on the wall, and watched him chuckling at it, I reacted rather aggressively.

'You old cynic,' I said. 'Just look at the advances in medicine over the last 50 years, and you've been at the forefront of it. You worked with Alexander Fleming on developing penicillin, you pioneered painless childbirth and played a major role in the development of safe contraception. You more than anyone should know how untrue that comment is.'

It is true that he swelled ever so slightly with pride at my remark, and it is also true that there was the trace of a smile in the corners of his mouth as he replied. 'Look,' he said, 'what medical activity have human beings been doing longer than any other, in fact for as long as there have been human beings on the planet?' I didn't know what he meant, and I said so.

'Being born,' he said with a hint of triumph in his voice. 'Yes, being born. And do you know how much we know about it? Nothing.

Absolutely nothing.' I challenged him, and he said, 'What is the best method of giving birth? Should you lie down, crouch, or sit in a pool? If we know so much about being born, how come there are still so many problems attached to it? If we know so much, why can't we guarantee to help people having problems? If the first Caesarian was performed two thousand years ago, how come it is still so difficult and risky? And how does the whole process actually work? Search me,' he said, this obstetrician who had delivered thousands of babies.

I wanted to argue with him, because what he was saying was so obviously over-simplistic, but later, thinking about it, I realised how much truth there was in it. And everything I have heard since about medicine has convinced me he was right. Bonnie's gynaecologist, for instance, made me her Number One fan when she said during one consultation, 'Stay away from people like me. Keep away from anyone wielding a scalpel.'

I thought of how hesitant the neurologist had been about pronouncing the diagnosis on Bonnie, and how interested he was in my descriptions of her behaviour.

Suchet's Law on Doctors and Medicine: The best doctors are the ones who admit they don't know.

How many times have you read in the papers, or heard on television, of a breakthrough in the treatment of breast cancer, or prostate cancer, of any other cancer, or, of course, Alzheimer's? Not more than once a day, probably. A former television critic of the *London Evening Standard*, Victor Lewis-Smith, once wrote, 'I measure the passing of time by how often TV news announces a cure for cancer.'

There isn't a cure for cancer. There probably never will be. The big advance is that it can now be treated. It is no longer an automatic death sentence. An oncologist told me at least a decade ago that now when he sat opposite a patient to break the news to them that they had cancer, the first thing he would say was, 'And this is what we are going to do to beat it.' Same with AIDS. Treatable. No longer an automatic death sentence.

If I am wrong, if I have let my cynicism run away with me, then why did Bonnie's brother Bob die of oesophageal cancer seven months ago? Or, more accurately, why did he get it in the first place?

We can treat disease, we can't stop it coming in the first place. But it's only a matter of time, I hear you say. You may be right. You may not be. Whatever. Don't hold your breath.

Rant over.

* * * *

In 1986 Bon and I had the most outrageous piece of good fortune, unbelievably good fortune. The opportunity arose for us to buy our flat. We couldn't believe our luck. We had fallen in love with that flat, our first real home. In the two weeks before moving in, I had decorated every room, and the long corridor. We had been in it for less than two years, but were happier than we had ever been.

Of course, I loved the block in which I had spent so many of my early years, but against all expectations Bonnie had come to love it too. It was – is – unique in London, in that it is held up by a tube station, one of the largest underground terminuses in the capital. It was, therefore, built and owned by London Transport. It has an interesting history, and I shall digress, with no apologies, to relate it.

Baker Street tube station is the oldest underground station in the world, opening in 1863. Some time in the early years of the last century, London Transport decided to build a hotel above the station, to accommodate the hordes of travellers they expected to flock into central London, once the Metropolitan line was extended out into the Chiltern Hills. The design was laid down, envisaging a large L-shaped building, stretching from close to Regent's Park on Baker Street, its corner at the junction of Baker Street and Marylebone Road, then running down to the next road junction (opposite the London Planetarium today). But at the outbreak of the First World War, work stopped. It was not taken up again until the early 1920s, by which time the decision had been made that the building would be a block of flats, not a hotel. The basic plan remained the same, which is why to this day the block is two long corridors in an L-shape with doors off them, just as in a hotel. It was opened in 1929 as an apartment block and named Chiltern Court after the Chiltern Hills, now served by the Metropolitan line.

Two plaques outside the main entrance today commemorate its most illustrious residents, the authors H.G. Wells and Arnold Bennett (who hated it). Bennett died in the block, and as he lay on his deathbed straw was put down on Marylebone Road to deaden the noise of the new steel-rimmed motorcar wheels.

During the Second World War, my grandfather the press photographer decided he needed a base in central London (he lived with my grandmother and mother in Stanmore), and my grandmother was dispatched to find somewhere suitable. She lighted upon Chiltern Court, and they moved in in late 1942. My parents married in early 1943 and moved in with them. Fourteen months later, I was born, and my parents took a flat of their own; two years later, my brother David was born; and seven years after that, my brother Peter. All the flats in the block were rented from London Transport. With a growing family, we moved out in the mid 1950s, but my parents moved back in 1979, and it was four years later that my mother secured the small flat on the top floor for Bonnie and me, and a year after that when we moved into the large flat which had seen Bonnie do that pirouette in the kitchen.

The fact that the flats were rented had saved us on my return from Washington, but as the months slipped by, we wanted something more secure. That's when the good Lord took pity on me and decided I needed a break. He told London Transport that they should sell Chiltern Court to the residents.

* * * *

2006 soon turned into a pretty difficult year. It had begun traumatically – Bon in for the brain tests, me starting at *Five News*, and then the diagnosis. As the year progressed, it became apparent to me that Bon's behaviour was altering, subtly at first, then more obviously. First to go was the computer. I realised she was no longer opening the laptop or doing any work on it. Next was her small electronic organiser, which in past years had been her Bible. Don't infer from this that she was in any way uncomfortable with electronic equipment, or regarded it as outside her sphere. It was Bonnie who, over a decade before, had helped me set templates when I began churning out my books on Beethoven, she who first taught herself, then me, to use the little organisers we both enjoyed so much. Slowly but surely, it all stopped.

Kitchen work stopped too. In past years she had cooked and cooked and cooked. How she loved cooking! She made the world's best pea and ham soup (taught by her mother, whose cookery book is still on our kitchen shelf), a stunning 'hamburger soup', so named by her boys who adored the self-invented concoction of minced beef, carrots, potatoes, and loads else (they were right, believe me), and a sherry trifle the thought of which even today sets my taste buds tingling. Some time in 2006 it slowed, then stopped. Effortlessly I took over. That needs rephrasing. Panic-stricken, having barely cooked in my life, I took over. But I was working full time at Channel Five and didn't get home till 8.30pm or later, too late to start cooking. Ready meals came to my rescue. Three minutes in the microwave, and you had a meal. I could get back from work, and we would be eating within 10 or 15 minutes. I was aware of the health issues – pre-prepared meant a lot of salt – so I persuaded Bon not to add extra. She was fine about it. To begin with, I asked her to dish up the food. She loved that. My heart broke to see how she enjoyed getting the portions exactly right. That didn't last long. I could soon see how she struggled to apportion the food properly. Without saying anything, I took over. She seemed relieved.

I was able to have lunch with Bon before going to work, so made sure there was a ready supply of pre-prepared salads in the fridge. Her appetite was diminishing, so we shared a single dish for dinner. We both began to lose weight. I was pleased for myself, but worried for Bonnie.

✲ ✲ ✲ ✲

Funny what money does to people. London Transport set a condition that they would only deal with a single company, not individual tenants, which meant the tenants of more than 150 flats had to come together, values had to be set on every flat, and the newly formed company had to agree on all terms. There was also a time limit. The sale had to go through by the end of 1987. There was one very attractive element. The law said that people renting their flats – in other words, sitting tenants – should be able to purchase their flat at a reduced price: for longer tenants at 50 per cent of the market value; for shorter ones, 75 per cent.

Instead of everyone walking round with a big smile on their face, this all led to enormous tension, even conflict. People who had been friends fell out. Why is your flat worth more than mine? Why isn't my flat worth more? Some people who had lived in the block for many years saw it as a chance to make a killing – buy the flat at 50 per cent, then sell immediately at a profit. Fractious meetings, arguments, and soon we were well into 1987. As for me, I simply smiled from ear to ear. Our flat was given its market value, in the low six figures, and I was told I was eligible to buy it at 75 per cent of that.

I knew it wouldn't be plain sailing. I needed a huge mortgage, and a 100 per cent loan for the down payment. First of all I went to see the deputy manager of our local NatWest, the bank I had been with for more than 20 years, and my father for twice as long as that.

Things got off to a perfect start. He told me he had seen me reporting on the television, and how pleased he was to be in a position to help us over such an important matter. There were pleasantries, and then he said

'Right, down to business. How can we be of help?' I gave it to him straight. The cost of the flat was £118,000. I had absolutely no capital, no savings, but Bonnie and I were both working. Our combined salaries were about £40,000. 'Shouldn't be a problem,' he said, 'let's look at the figures.'

He pulled an ominously large calculator towards him, and began tapping. He asked me what my outgoings were. I told him I was paying roughly half my net income in child support, and he frowned ominously. More tapping. Finally, a heavy tap on the equals key, his eyebrows shot up, and he leaned back in his chair. 'The figures don't really add up, do they? Have you ever considered moving out to the country?'

I was too stunned to speak. I can't remember what was said next, or who said it. I just remember us finding ourselves outside his office, on the landing, the door closed behind us.

I would have given up at that stage, but Bon insisted that we try the Midland Bank right underneath Chiltern Court. She had to use all her efforts at persuasion because I didn't want to put myself through another humiliating session. As it turned out, this was quite different.

We sat opposite the manager, a nice man with a kindly smile by the name of Peter Thorne. I was stony-faced, allowing Bonnie to do most of the talking. 'Well,' he said, 'let's have a look at the figures.' Tap tap tap, and the inevitable words, 'Mmm, there is a bit of a problem, the figures don't really add up. You wouldn't be able to meet the monthly payments on a 100 per cent mortgage.' I was in such a depression that I couldn't speak. There was no fight in me. Figures were figures.

He looked from Bonnie to me, and back again, up at the ceiling, then down again with a smile of triumph on his face. 'We'll make this work for you. We can't let this opportunity go. I know what we'll do. You're getting your flat at 75 per cent of the market value, is that right?' I nodded. 'So you're saving 25 per cent. We'll call that 25 per cent the deposit, which means you've already paid it, and we'll give you a mortgage on the rest. How does that sound?'

It's not often you want to kiss a bank manager. I moved my account immediately to the Midland, later HSBC, and Bonnie and I have banked there ever since. Many years later, Peter Thorne, now retired, asked if I would give a music talk in Southend, where he and his wife lived. 'Just tell me where and when, and I'll be there.'

Soon after these interviews, I received a letter from the manager of NatWest expressing his sadness that I was leaving the bank. In my reply I told him exactly why, and I can remember quoting his deputy's suggestion about us moving to the country, and writing, 'This wins the 1987 Least Helpful Suggestion of the Year Award'.

I have been back into the NatWest building many times with Bon over the years. It is a Pizza Express.

* * * *

I was worried about my work at Channel Five. Sooner or later, I feared, the effect of the strain I was under would begin to show. I had told Chris Shaw, the man who had hired me, about Bonnie, and I also told three key people in the newsroom, including the editor. I felt they should know. What if it all got on top of me? What if, less dramatically, I began to make the odd mistake or two on air? I had been a television newscaster for 20 years, and right up until the very last bulletin I used to get nervous. It is an overwhelmingly big job. You are carrying the work of a hundred people on your shoulders, you are going into millions of living rooms. You need to be at the top of your game, razor sharp. The one thing you don't need, in any form whatsoever, is pressure from outside. I had that, in spades.

Bonnie's confusion was beginning to become more evident. A sentence would come out which made perfect sense, but which bore no relation to reality. Dementia was progressing, inexorably.

I told no one outside the immediate family about the diagnosis, with the few exceptions at Channel Five. All five boys knew, as well as my brothers, and Bonnie's family in America. That was it. No one else. There was no need, yet. I cut several friends loose, without explanation. I simply turned down invitations. Sooner or later, I imagined, I would have to say something more publicly, if only to stop persistent enquiries, but for the moment that could wait. I began to look slightly less far ahead. No more long-term planning. Who could tell what lay ahead next year, next month, next week, tomorrow?

* * * *

1986 really was an *annus mirabilis.* I progressed from reporter to newscaster, which was to change my career for ever (though I didn't know it at the time), we were offered our flat to buy, and Bonnie landed the job of a lifetime. But first, there was the job *not* of a lifetime.

She had been temping, and pretty grim it had been. She signed up with several agencies, and plodded off to do some lowly secretarial tasks. I told her to apply for something more permanent, but she said no, she had to work her way in, get experience, so she would know what to look for.

One day she said she was going for an interview with a small firm of accountants run by two men who needed a full-time secretary. I remember she wore the same pink suede suit I had helped her out of in New York. She looked every inch the senior executive. She came home saying the interview had gone very well, but she looked a little uneasy. One of the men, she said, had made her feel uncomfortable.

She got the job, of course, and pretty much hated it from Day One. This one man had clearly fallen in love with her (no surprise there). She had taken an immediate dislike to him. She found him oily and ingratiating, and his greasy hair needed an encounter with a shampoo bottle. He had absolutely no idea how to talk to her, she said. Innuendos, suggestions, never explicit, trying to ingratiate himself with her. He was also a know-all. Mention any topic, from politics to music, via Greek islands, nuclear physics, and space technology, and he always knew about it, enough at least to sound impressive for about a nanosecond.

One day she came home, slammed her briefcase down in disgust, and said, 'You're not going to believe this. On the wall above his desk, there's a calendar with pictures of pretty English villages. Behind it, he's got a *Playboy* calendar. Eeeuugh!'

She contacted the agency that had sent her for the job and said she didn't like it, and if anything better came along she would like them to tell her. It didn't, for quite a long time, probably because the agency considered that since she had a full-time job, like it or not, she was off their books. Then one day they called her and said they knew of a vacancy at a company, but it was rather weird. Several of their clients had gone for interview, but it seemed rather secretive. They couldn't say exactly what the job was. All they knew was they hadn't been offered it. Would Bonnie like to go along? I said no immediately. Sounded thoroughly dodgy, and I didn't want a repeat of Mr Oily Accountant. Bon said, Why not? Can't hurt. I'll go.

I am nothing if not an over-protective paranoid male (as most men with beautiful wives probably are). The interview was at an address just the other side of Oxford Street. I decided to drive Bon there. I parked in a side road and walked her across to the building. I then sat in the car, trying to concentrate on the *Times* crossword.

Half an hour went by, then an hour, then an hour-and-a-half. Was it a good sign? Certainly at the hour mark, but by the hour-and-a-half mark mild panic was beginning to set in. There was the added thought that even if it was going well, what if it was a thoroughly dubious job? I had images of Bonnie being trafficked to the Middle East. I am usually pretty good at the *Times* crossword. I can guarantee to solve at least three clues, on a good day four or even five. If I remember rightly, on this occasion my tally stood at two.

Finally I saw her emerge, intact, with a quizzical smile on her face. I dashed across the road, took her by the arm and walked her back to the car. 'How are you? Was it OK?' She was smiling and said, 'It went so well.' 'That's wonderful,' I said, convinced she was about to tell me she needed to get on a plane to Saudi Arabia.

I didn't want her to face a barrage of questions, so I waited for her to speak. All she said was 'I'll tell you more when we get home.' OK, fine, I can wait, but she flies to bloody Saudi Arabia over my dead body.

We got into the flat, put the kettle on, made tea, and sat together in the sitting room. 'Tell me everything,' I said. 'Well, there's not much to tell, really. There were two men, really nice guys. They said they were part of a large multi-national company that was also a charitable foundation, with one man, an American, at its head. He's apparently pretty wealthy. This man sort of travels the world, but he wants to establish a base in London, and he needs a PA here. That's what the job is. The one thing they were really interested in, seemed really keen on, was that I went to Cornell University.' I asked where else the company had offices. 'They said New York, San Francisco, Dublin, Bermuda, I think, and now London.'

'Hah, dodgy financial dealings,' I said knowingly. 'There's no way you're going to get involved in that.' 'No,' she said, 'it's not like that, I'm sure. It all sounds totally genuine.' 'Well who is this guy, this American, and what's the name of the company?' A look of slight anxiety came over her face. 'That's the thing. I don't know. They said at this stage they would rather not tell me.' 'I know exactly what's going on,' I said. 'There is no such company. There is no such man. It's all a front. I know about stuff like this. I'm a journalist. I've heard about dodgy dealings like this. Anyway, you are too straight for them, they'll have realised that. You won't hear from them again, I bet you. And that top man who wants a PA. He doesn't exist, believe me.'

'I think he does,' she said. 'He's going to ring me from New York in about an hour.'

* * * *

Things were happening that were a real worry. In August 2006, six months after the diagnosis (I now think of our lives as pre-diagnosis and post-diagnosis), Bonnie lost her watch, a rather lovely gold Cartier that I had bought her many years before. We were down in France, and on the morning of our departure she said she couldn't find it.

I was used to her being unable to find things, and either I would manage to locate the missing object or it would turn up in the fullness of time. This time, I told her I knew where it was – I had seen it on her dressing table in our bedroom upstairs. But it was no longer there. She searched high and low, so did I, no luck, and we came home without it.

Over the following months, I kept an eye out for it, but it really was nowhere to be found. I became convinced it had gone, that somehow I had swept it into the wastepaper basket beside the dressing table and thrown it out with the rubbish. After a year I decided it had gone forever and bought her a new watch, a Longines this time to match the Longines she had bought me, also many years before.

Some months later I was sitting on the terrace at our French house, immersed in a book. Suddenly she was beside me and she said, 'Look, I have found your watch.' I grunted something, then glanced at my wrist and saw my watch. Odd. I looked at her wrist, and there was the Longines I had bought her. On her right wrist was the Cartier.

I yelped with delight. 'Your watch! You've found it!' She looked confused. 'It's *your* watch,' she said. 'Darling!' I ploughed happily on, 'that's your watch, the one you lost over a year ago!' 'Oh good, that means we've found it,' she said. 'It certainly does. Where did you find it? Come on, tell me, where has it been hiding all this time?' I knew as soon as I said it that it was a mistake. The look of confusion on her face intensified. She shook her head. I wasn't going to give up. 'Come upstairs with me,' I said, 'to the bedroom, then you can show me where you found it.' We went upstairs, but yes, you've guessed it. Blank.

I realised there was no point in pressing it. She simply didn't remember. I don't know to this day where she found it.

* * * *

The phone went in the flat, right on cue. I watched Bon answering it, knowing she wouldn't mind. It was a remarkably brief conversation, though conversation is hardly the right word. She smiled throughout, nodding, saying yes over and over again, putting the phone down in probably not much more than a minute.

I gaped at her in expectation. The smile was still on her face, and she said, 'Strange. He didn't ask me anything. He just told me a bit about himself. He said he had been to Cornell, like me.' 'Did he offer you the job?' I asked, ever keen to cut through the subtleties. 'Well, no. He just assumed I had got it. He said he looked forward to meeting me in the office next week, when he's back.'

I couldn't quell suspicion, mistrust, concern, worry. What was my Bonnie getting herself into? I need not have worried. For the next 15 years, Bon was PA to one of the most remarkable men I have ever met.

His name is Charles Feeney, known universally as Chuck. He is one of the wealthiest men in the world, and definitely *the* most modest. He made his money selling duty-free goods. There is a legend, part true at least, that in his early days he set up a table at Hawaii airport, loaded with duty-free, and slept under it, waiting for the planes to land. By the 1980s, he had a personal fortune of several hundred million dollars, and nobody knew who he was. That was the way he wanted it. He had only one ambition – to give away his fortune before he died. In effect, that was impossible, because he couldn't stop the money from his company, Duty Free Shoppers, coming in. But he has had a damn good try.

As a first generation Irish-American, he enrolled at Cornell University to study hotel management. His parents couldn't afford the fees, so to try and make ends meet he made sandwiches in the early morning and sold them to students at lunchtime, wearing a billboard front and back advertising himself as Sandwich Man (a nickname still used by those who go back that far). In gratitude for the education Cornell gave him, he has endowed the university with a fortune, allowing them to build a new hotel school. The university asked permission to name the school after him. Horror upon horror! That was not his way; anonymity was what he wanted. In honour of his Irish heritage, he has donated a fortune to the University of Limerick too.

When Bonnie took me to meet him for the first time, she warned me to brace myself. 'Don't worry,' I said, 'I'm used to meeting important and successful people.' Hadn't I interviewed President Reagan and Prime Minister Thatcher? 'No,' she said, 'that's not what I mean. You won't believe it's him. He won't talk much. He won't be what you expect.'

She was right. A suit that had seen better days, shoes that had that look of being so comfortable he probably hadn't taken them off for years, looking up from heavily lidded eyes that betrayed a sense of insecurity, of not belonging, feeling out of place, a voice surprisingly high-pitched, uttering short words at machine-gun speed, as if to hide the unavoidable New Jersey accent with Irish twinge. I looked at him slightly tongue-tied (unusual, yes). He couldn't wait to get away and back to work. 'Bonnie, ah, yeah, very good,' is about all I can remember from the first conversation.

She soon became his indispensable right-hand 'man'. A steady stream of callers from all over the world would hear the words, 'Speak to Bonnie, she knows what I'm doing.'

For 15 years, Bonnie was at the heart of this global company, and at the side of this man, as his foundation supervised the giving away of many millions of dollars to educational enterprises. She ran his life – booked his flights (always economy class), arranged accommodation (he had no permanent address), booked restaurants. He came to rely on her calm, utterly dedicated efficiency.

In the 1990s Chuck became involved in the Northern Ireland peace process, in an informal and private capacity. As a journalist, I knew this was a story – American billionaire attempts to bring peace to the troubled province. Bon said to me, You won't tell anyone, will you? As if I would. A scoop at the risk of upsetting my Bonnie? Don't be silly, it was never an option.

Bon retired in 2001, to coincide with her 60th birthday. Chuck gave her an amazing send-off at a hotel he had built outside Limerick. Weeks before, Bon told me she was terrified about having to make a speech, and would I help her? *Would I?* I let her work out what she wanted to say, then in the bridal suite of the hotel I rehearsed her, encouraging her to repeat the speech out loud several times (a technique I always use myself). At first embarrassed, shy, and speaking at minus zero decibels, slowly she gained in confidence, until she could speak out loud with a smile permanently on her face.

Her speech was a triumph. When we retired to the suite at the end of an unforgettable evening, I congratulated her again and again. 'Your speech was the highlight,' I said, 'you did so well.' 'I learned from the master,' she said. I know, I know, I didn't need to relate that. But it was such a lovely compliment, so genuinely delivered, and I believe it says more about her utterly giving character than it does about me. Thus ended a wonderful and fulfilling era of her life, and I was proud to have shared in it.

Chuck, as I write this, is nearing 80 years of age. He and his wife divide their time between apartments in San Francisco and Sydney – still no permanent home. When they pass through London, they are always in touch. Chuck's health is not too good, and he is, predictably, finding it hard to let go. A couple of years ago an authorised biography of him was published, entitled *The Billionaire Who Wasn't*. Authorised, maybe, but you'd better not mention it to him. He'll mumble, embarrassed, and change the subject.

* * * *

A year after diagnosis, I take Bonnie for a cognitive test at the National Neurological Hospital. The usual questions, and always 'spell world backwards'. Her score has dropped dramatically. I am not really surprised. What *does* surprise me is she sits through it, patiently answering the questions, or failing to, without once asking me what this is all about, and why she is having to do it.

It really is as if this wretched disease might have one redeeming quality. It is protecting Bonnie from understanding what is happening to her.

As for me, when we get home I quietly cry, secretly in another room. I realise I am losing my Bonnie, slowly but unstoppably.

Chapter 6

I had an e-mail via my website a few months ago from a name from the past. At first I had trouble remembering who it was. It said simply we had met at La Valouze almost 20 years before, and he had some interesting information about him and Sharon. Signed Bob.

I had to read it several times, but slowly the distant and forgotten past filtered through into my now much more aged brain. In spring 1989 Bon said to me she wanted to fulfill a long-standing ambition to learn French. I can't now remember whose idea it was, but we came up with a plan to go to France for our summer holiday, two weeks, and enroll in a French language course somewhere. Again, it is too long ago to recall how we researched it (so easy today, on the internet), but we found two places – one was on the French Riviera, near Cannes, a modern-looking building in a relatively busy street 100 metres or so from the beach, the other a château in the Dordogne by the name of La Valouze. We chose the château, little suspecting it would lead to a decision that would change our lives.

Shortly before leaving for France, in early August, I received a call in the flat from the Frenchman who ran the course (a former member of the French Foreign Legion, the brochure said enticingly). Speaking in English, he asked why my wife had enrolled in the language course, but I hadn't. 'You will sit all day in your chalet,' he said. 'That's fine,' I replied, 'I'll bring lots of books to read.' 'But why not take the course? If you do not understand French, you will learn. If you do, you will improve.' 'I really …' He suddenly switched to French, asking me if I spoke the language. Calmly, and I must admit rather suavely, I switched easily into French, explaining that I had lived in Paris for the best part of two years, had been a Reuters correspondent on the streets of the city during *les événements* of 1968, had covered the resignation of President de Gaulle, and so on. That brought the conversation to an end.

We had one further decision to make. The course was a week, our holiday was for two. How should we spend the second week? I had an idea. Two things had recently happened. I had read an article in the *Sunday Times Magazine* about Gascony in south-west France, home of the Musketeers, utterly beautiful and unexplored. There were plenty of Brits to the north in Dordogne and to the south in the Basque region, but not in Gascony. The area was rich in history, ruled by the English before and during the Hundred Years' War, pillaged by the Black Prince, redolent with *bastides*, small fortified towns built by both the French and English during that long war. 'Explore the white roads,' the article said, referring to the Michelin map. The second thing was that I had just read *The Three Musketeers*. I became instantly fascinated with Gascony – and Gascons, larger than life, jovial, flamboyant, posturing, fighters not of bulls but young heifers who are restrained by ropes with no weapons used, champion consumers of the local speciality, Armagnac. In other words, Musketeers. Not for nothing is the French word for exaggeration *gasconard*.

'Why don't we hire a car and tour Gascony for the second week?' 'Nice idea,' Bon said.

And so in August 1989 we arrived one swelteringly hot afternoon at the Château La Valouze, in the heart of Dordogne. We met around a dozen fellow Brits who had enrolled, and to be honest I can remember none of them, except two. One was an Irishman from Dublin named Bob, who was a bit older than the rest of us (probably in his early to mid fifties), and an extraordinarily glamorous blonde by the name of Sharon. Bob, he later told us, was a senior executive with Norwich Union who had just been appointed Head of Europe, and so needed to learn French.

He was a naturally funny man, who had most of us in stitches much of the time with his quips. He was hopeless at French, and he, the teachers, in fact most of us, realised pretty quickly that a year of lessons would have had little impact, let alone a week. He was able to laugh at this, feigning panic that he would lose the promotion. Sharon hailed from southern England and, like Bonnie, had come to learn French because it was something she'd always wanted to do. No matter how hot the weather, no matter how tattily clothed many of us were, Sharon always looked immaculate, usually in a white dress, with glorious jewellery that caught the sun, surrounding her in shafts of light that illuminated her blonde hair and light skin. I nicknamed her 'Glam Lady'. Both Bob and Sharon were married, but had left their spouses at home and embarked alone on the serious task of learning French.

From the moment he set eyes on her, Bob fell head over heels in love with Sharon. You didn't need to be an Einstein to work this out. Bob told us all, including Sharon. With the wonderful lilt of an Irish accent in his voice, and sparkles of laughter in his eyes, he couldn't stop talking about how he had been smitten. His French, as I said, was hopeless, so hopeless that he told the teachers there was only one sentence he wanted to perfect, so he could say it to Sharon in French, and that was 'Will you go to bed with me?' – and he only finally got it right as he left at the end of the course.

It was a week of fun and laughter, with no one taking themselves – or the task at hand – too seriously. The teachers roped me in to take some classes and I took to the task with gusto. In one lesson there was a suitcase full of items of clothing, which the students had to identify in French. I took slightly dubious delight in selecting the briefest of shorts for Sharon to identify, then told her, in French, to put them on her head.

On the final evening there was a grand party, in which we all had to sing French songs. Bob, senior international insurance executive, Chinese wig with pigtails on his head, sang his heart out, with Sharon kneeling at his feet holding up the sheet of lyrics for him to read. He introduced her as 'my groupie'.

Fond farewells, and we all went our separate ways. To begin our second week, the tour of Gascony, I had booked a room for a single night in a small hotel in a village at the foot of the Pyrenees. Not exactly Gascony, but I thought a little mountain air would be welcome after the stifling heat of Dordogne. From there we would motor north to the Atlantic coast (I had already selected a hotel for night two), and then inland to the town of Auch, the capital of Gascony. Don't worry about a thing, I said to Bon, I've got it all worked out.

We arrived at the hotel in the Pyrenees at around five in the afternoon, took one look at it and drove on. It didn't look up to much, and after the grandiloquent luxury of La Valouze, I wanted to keep the standards up for Bon. She said fine, whatever you think, but it's nearly five, we don't want to get stuck with nowhere to stay. Of course not, I said, don't worry, I've got it under control.

Up into the mountains and into a café, where we had a cup of tea and I asked if I could use the telephone. I called the hotel where we were going to stay for the second night and told them I would like to book a room for tonight. '*Complet. Désolé,*' was the response. All right, no problem, we will drive to the coast. Hotels by the score, I told Bon reassuringly. To the coast we drove, to the town of Capbreton. It was teeming. The seafront was bristling with hotels. A little beneath the standard I wanted, but it was six o'clock or thereabouts, and it was only for one night after all.

First hotel '*complet*', second hotel '*complet*', third hotel '*complet*' – and I began to panic. 'Don't tell me there isn't a single room in this entire town?' I said in exasperation. Bon should of course have replied, 'Did it not occur to you, Monsieur le Francophile, who knows everything there is to know about the French and their habits on account of how you used to live and work here, that the south of France in August might just be ever so slightly crowded, *imbécile*?' But she did not. 'Why don't we go to the tourist office?' she suggested quietly, 'they'll know which hotels have rooms.' 'No, no,' I said masterfully, 'what we'll do is … we'll … I know, we'll go to the tourist office.' 'Good idea,' she said.

'We need a room for tonight, please, Mademoiselle.' *'Aucun problème,'* and she turned to the shelf behind her and gathered up several sheets of paper. I looked at Bon in triumph. 'Right, the best for you is 'ere, you must go down zees road, turn right 'ere, and at the end is ze house. They have one small room. Zere is bed and breakfast, but no breakfast, because ze man, ees wife is ill. It will cost you 200 francs [around £20].'

'Erm … I was thinking more in terms of a three-star hotel with a private suite and swimming pool.'

She looked at me as if I was completely mad. 'Nothing,' she said, 'zere is nothing,' and shook her head. 'All right,' I said resignedly, 'we'll go to the bed and –' 'Only 90 kilometres away. You would need to drive for two hours.' 'You mean, there is a luxury hotel?' 'Not near. You must drive –' 'Would you please call them and ask them if they have a large double, a suite even?' She vanished into the office. I could hear the conversation. *'Oui, oui, ils vont arriver vers vingt heures et demi, vingt et une heures. Merci!'*

I drove slightly too fast, zipping through quaint stone villages faster than they deserved. Around two hours later, on the ring road of the town of Mont-de-Marsan, rising oasis-like in the middle of a parched desert, was a brilliantly white hotel, the appropriate name of 'La Renaissance' beckoning invitingly. We walked in, travel-weary and tired. The hall was tiled and cool, there was a faint smell of fresh paint, and a stronger aroma of cooking. I turned and smiled at Bonnie. They offered us the choice of a double room or a suite. It was not a difficult decision.

* * * *

Bonnie's cousin Carol came to visit us in late April 2007. Bonnie and Carol grew up like sisters. It was over a year since the diagnosis, and the effects were more self-evident with every passing month. Carol hadn't seen Bon for a while, so you can imagine how shocked she was. Little did she – or I – know what was in store.

Looking back on it now, maybe it wasn't such a big deal, but at the time … We all went down to France. There was one precaution I was now taking every time we travelled. On arrival at the airport, as soon as we were through passport control, I took Bonnie's passport from her and kept it in my briefcase. She didn't like me doing it, she said she wasn't a child, but she acquiesced. This had begun after the summer of 2003, when on leaving France she had been unable to find her passport. Really unable. I said I would look. I couldn't find it either. I searched everywhere, high and low, but it was nowhere. We had no option but to go to the airport without her passport. It involved reporting to the airport police, who said we would have to go into the town to the main police station, which would mean abandoning travelling home for at least a day, maybe more. Bonnie looked at the officer sadly. He shrugged, looked at her again, and said on this occasion he would make an exception, then stamped the necessary papers for us, which allowed us to board the flight. Once home, Bonnie applied for a new passport. A year later we found the old passport, which she had hidden inside a thick pullover at the back of a clothes drawer to keep it safe.

We stayed in France for 10 days. I was heavily stuck into writing a book on Beethoven. Carol chatted to Bonnie as much as she could, spent every minute with her she could. We had a good time. We were due to return to London on an early flight on Wednesday in the first week of May. I had a ticket that evening, as guest of the Royal Academy of Music, at the newly refurbished Royal Festival Hall.

We got up early, snatched a quick breakfast, and I went into my well-rehearsed 'turn things off and close the shutters' routine. Finally, all three of us were ready to leave. I checked the inner zipped pocket of my brief-case for our passports. Mine was there, but not Bonnie's. Odd (again). I remembered taking the passport from her at Pau airport and putting it with mine into that pocket and zipping it closed. I looked again, and again, and again, in all the other pockets, I tipped the whole bag out. No sign of Bonnie's passport.

I felt the stirrings of panic. I ran upstairs, checked surfaces and drawers, then clothes pockets. Nothing. I ran downstairs, checked drawers, cupboards, coat pockets, nothing. The stirrings matured into pure panic. Carol was as stunned as I was. 'But I saw you take it from Bonnie at the airport and put it into your briefcase,' she said. I nodded. It was routine. But it was not there now.

For the next half hour, with time ticking ominously away, I turned the house upside down. Panic had now consumed me, because I knew that what I was doing was futile. I was simply re-searching in areas I had already searched.

Finally I admitted defeat. I slumped into a kitchen chair. 'I have a touch of the *déjà vu*,' I said. 'We will have to go to the airport, report to the police, then almost certainly have to go into the town to the main police station. We won't be able to travel today. I'll have to telephone the Academy. I don't know what …'

Bonnie suddenly said, 'Well, I have found mine. What about yours?' And she was waving her passport triumphantly in the air. Carol and I looked at each other. The blood flowed back into my face. We rushed out to the car and left for the airport.

Like the watch, I don't know to this day where that passport had been or how it got there.

The hotel was indeed newly built, fresh paint everywhere, new furnishings, and we were among its first guests. It was idyllic. For Bonnie and me, it was like a second honeymoon. The chef came and chatted to us: was the food all right, what did we think, try this wine, now that one. The weather was hot and seductive, the swimming pool cool and inviting. It was mid-August, and we spent the first three days sitting by the pool, reading, taking a dip to cool off, summer salads and chilled wine for lunch, duck – in all its forms, the staple diet of Gascony – and local red wine for dinner. I read a biography of Napoleon by Vincent Cronin.

I was – am – a Francophile, unreconstructed. Put it down to my early years as a journalist in Paris. I fell in love with France and the French, and am still in love. Their language, culture, history, their food and wine, everything. I have a French surname, that borne by a distinguished Marshal in Napoleon's army, elevated to the dukedom by him, the name carved on the Arc de Triomphe, and also given to one of the *grands boulevards* that surround Paris. It pains me to reveal he is not my ancestor, my name is not French but the Frenchification of a Lithuanian name, and I have not a drop of French blood in my veins. So what? I still adore the country. From my years in Paris I had always harboured a secret fantasy that one day, maybe, I would have a home in France. An impossible dream, but you never know.

On Day Four, I said to Bon, Why don't we do what that *Sunday Times* article said and explore the white roads? She agreed. I can't remember exactly where we drove, but one thing I do remember – I had never seen so many old houses, practically ruins, all with crude hand-painted signs saying *À Vendre*. I became somewhat mesmerised by this. So many old houses for sale, I said to Bon, such a pity to see them in such disrepair. The germ of an idea formed in my mind, but I said nothing. Impossible. Ridiculous. Put it right out of your mind, John.

The next day, Friday 18th August, we took to the white roads again. Those houses hadn't gone away. I commented on it again, and this time we stopped once or twice and walked round a derelict building or two. Laughingly we joked about what fun it would be to do one up. Just a joke. Nothing serious.

It was Bonnie – it really was – who said at one point around noon, 'Funny, all the signs have a name on them, the same name, Aire something. Do you think it is an estate agent?' I consulted the map. 'No, it's the nearest big town, Aire-sur-l'Adour. Look.' I showed her the map. She said – really, it was she who said it, not me – 'Why don't we go there for lunch?' 'Good idea,' I said, 'I'm starving.'

We arrived in Aire and parked the car by the river. There was a café close by, but we decided – both of us – to have a little stroll, stretch our legs, before lunch. We sauntered up the main street of the town, nice-looking little shops, more cafés, people sitting and having lunch, chatting, enjoying the hot August sun. Halfway down the street, on the corner, was a small estate agent. Bonnie said, 'Let's look in the window.' Why not? No harm done. There was a glass cabinet with badly taken Polaroid photos in it. 'Look, that one,' she said, 'something like that, don't you think?' I stared at a poorly composed picture of a lot of mud, beyond it a high hangar on rickety legs, a drab barely visible building attached to it, with a long barn in an L-shape which looked about to fall down. To this city boy, it was not a pretty sight.

'Yes, well,' I muttered, feet turning instantly cold, foolish fantasies dying on the spot, 'let's go and have lunch.' 'Let's go in,' she said, 'come on, just for fun.' I had a sinking feeling in my stomach, instantly relieved when we found the door locked, the office closed for lunch.

We sat outside the café down by the river and ordered sandwiches as only the French can make them – thick crusty baguettes sliced down the middle with filling. Bon ordered cheese and I annoyingly asked the waiter what the local speciality was. Ham, from Bayonne, he said, nodding in the general direction of the coast. That was for me. A chilled *panaché* (I had learned in Paris that the verb *panacher*, to mix, was used on its own in the past participle to mean shandy) was the perfect complement.

We sat marveling at how anywhere in France, between noon and two o'clock, everything was shut, everyone at lunch (at least, that's how it was in 1989). At the end of the meal, I said – yes, this time it was me, and I can't for the life of me understand what made me say it, because I had not the slightest intention of taking things even the next infinitesimal step further – 'Shall we go back to that estate agent, see if it is open?' 'Yes, let's,' said Bon. And we did.

She pointed at that photo again and said, 'That one. That's the one.' I pushed at the door and in we went, to be met by a woman behind a desk whose face, when she heard my accent, lit up like a light bulb. Haltingly, for Paris had been two decades before and the subject matter was new to me, I explained that we were English tourists, that we were most emphatically not looking for a house, that we had no intention whatsoever of buying a house (rendered less sophisticatedly into French as *Acheter … non, non, non*, with much shaking of the head), but my wife (finger pointing accusingly at Bon) had seen a photo in the window, and we were just wondering …

She stood up and opened the window panel in towards her and Bon pointed again at *that* photo. '*Non, non*,' the woman said, making disapproving clucking noises with her tongue, 'not that one, you don't want to see that one. I have something much better.' She opened a folder and took out a photo of a small town house. 'Zees one,' switching into English, 'vairy nice. Ozzer one,' she wrinkled her nose. '*Venez*. I will show you.' I started to explain that we didn't want to see anywhere, we just wanted an idea of price so we could go away and have a chat about it, and could she please tell us about this one, as I pointed again at the photo Bon had first noticed.

'You will see zem bose. Zere is no problem.' I protested again, but she had picked up a telephone and was soon talking at a zillion kilometres an hour. I picked up the gist of it. She was arranging for us to see one of the houses. A slight feeling of dread was brewing up in my stomach. She smiled and pointed at the Bon photo. 'Zees one will we see. I 'ave arranged. But first, come, I show you ozzer one.' Before I could say another word, she had ushered us out of the office and was locking the door behind her.

I sat in the front of the car with her, Bon behind, as she asked us where we were staying, how long we had been in the area, did we like it, where did we live in England, and I was struggling to keep up. I was also striving to make up my mind about how we were going to extricate ourselves from this rather perilous situation. Finally we arrived in the main square of a small village. She pointed at a singularly unprepossessing townhouse. As we walked towards it, I saw a net curtain twitch in an adjoining house and a suspicious female face peer out. My mind was made up before we even stepped inside the empty house. '*Non*,' I said, and she nodded, as if it had come as no real shock to her. '*Aucun problème*. Now I show you ozzer one.'

We drove for a good 10 minutes or so, finally up a rather long hill, turned right onto a main road, and left into a lane which dog-legged round to the right. Immediately in front of us stood a small cottage in a dilapidated state. 'Tch, tch,' she clucked, waving her index finger, 'not zees one, but … zees one.' She stopped the car, we got out and found ourselves looking at the Polaroid photo Bon had first pointed at.

It was large, spacious, set in its own land, the house crying out to be renovated. She took us through the front door. The smell of damp was everywhere. The rooms were small, with wallpaper hanging down in strips. The kitchen was long and narrow, a small window and single dirty sink. We stepped out of the kitchen onto earth, where a bathroom and toilet, *circa* 1930, stood forlornly. To our right was the huge barn set in an L-shape to the house, but it was too dangerous to go in, because animals had been kept there and it was now structurally unsound. Into the main sitting room, the *séjour*, larger than the other rooms, with a door out to the back. She opened this door, we stepped outside, and Bon let out a gasp. 'Look! Just look!' she said, 'the view. It's beautiful.' We were gazing across about an acre of rough ground that stretched off to the left and belonged to the house, but which the agent explained was for sale separately, to a deep valley which fell, then rose again in the distance as far as the eye could see. The landscape was a thousand different shades of green, and there was a deafening din of birds.

I, city boy, marveled at the tranquility of it all. I turned to Bonnie. She was standing there, just gazing into the distance. She turned to me and I could see tears of happiness in her eyes. I think I said something crass like 'Not exactly Baker Street, is it?'

I smiled at the woman, thanked her, and said the house was really lovely, and we would like to go now and have a big think. She nodded and led us back out of the front door. In the few seconds it took us to emerge, I began to wonder *What if?* but just as swiftly put it out of my mind. I was woken from my reverie by the woman exclaiming, *'Aaah! Monsieur! Voilà! Ça va?'*

A man of around my age, about my height, with tight curly black hair, was walking towards us. We shook hands all round, in the French style, and he introduced himself. 'Jean-Pierre,' he said, smiling broadly.

Two social workers from Central and North West London NHS came to the flat. One sat with Bon, while the other explained the help that was available out there for me. 'You have access to an Admiral Nurse,' she said. I can't remember exactly what I said, but I think it was something along the lines of, 'I don't think I do. I never did National Service, and I was certainly never in the navy.'

Patiently she explained to me that Admiral Nurses were specially trained mental health nurses, whose role was to help all those affected by dementia, especially carers. They had been established by a family of which the patriarch had died with dementia. The family had realised that although there was medical help for him, there was no help or advice for them, the carers, yet it was on them, his wife in particular, that the greatest burden fell. They decided to do something about it, and so Admiral Nurses came into being, named after the old man, who was known as Admiral Joe for his love of sailing.

She also explained, somewhat to my horror, that very few NHS Trusts in the country provide Admiral Nurses. 'It all depends on where you live,' she said. 'You're lucky. Westminster comes under Central and

North West London, and the local NHS Trust provides Admiral Nurses. In fact, they were the first in the country to do so.'

Still I said, Thank you very much, but I don't need that kind of help. Yes, Bonnie was clearly becoming more forgetful, but it was nothing I couldn't handle without a bit of effort. Also the word 'nurse' made it all sound so medical. So I took it no further. Then came the trip to France and the passport incident. I told Carol about Admiral Nurses. She said I would be stupid not to follow up on it. 'You need help,' she said, 'more than you think.'

I made a phone call, and that was how Ian Weatherhead, Admiral Nurse, came into my life.

It is probably not an exaggeration to say that in the months and years to come, Ian saved my life. In our sessions, he not only helped me to understand Bonnie's behaviour, but more importantly he helped me to understand my own. He taught me that I am allowed to have an off day, that I am allowed to lose my temper, that my behaviour – unusual, even bizarre, though it may appear to me – is normal. I have learned that there is nothing a carer wants to hear more than that the way they are behaving is normal.

He explained to me, too, that I was in mourning, going through the grieving process, for someone who was actually still physically there. It was a blinding revelation. Those dark moments when the tears suddenly come, when the memories come back that I can no longer share. It's a bereavement, and yet the person you are in mourning for is still there.

How do you cope with that alone? The short answer, as I learned, is you cannot.

* * * *

The estate agent hung back and Jean-Pierre took over. He led us round the house again, but this time pointing out what we could do with it. This wall down to create a huge *séjour*, this wall down to open up the kitchen. He took us into the perilously standing barn, even upstairs where he advised against testing the floorboards. Then into the dirty, dusty, dark attic. 'This could be a magnificent bedroom,' he said, 'just raise the roof, build the walls up, put big windows in.' I shook my head. Impossible, impractical. Something caught my eye, standing on the low sill of the single tiny window. I picked it up – a dirty dusty statuette of the Virgin Mary. Jean-Pierre smiled. 'Take it. It will bring you luck.'

Standing at the top of a single small flight of rotting stairs, I said 'Look, we are foreigners, and I only get a few weeks' holiday a year.' He interrupted. 'We would look after everything for you. When the sun shines, my wife will open the windows; when it rains, she will close them. It could all be magnificent,' he said. I blanched. But it would take years, I said. *'Petit à petit,'* he said.

He explained that the house had been in his family for many generations, maybe 200 years, and that he had been born in it. In the late 1940s, his father had bought another house just 100 metres or so up the road, which had much more space for farm equipment, and where the family still lived. Ever since, he had rented this house out, but now they had decided to sell it. Come, I will show you something, he said.

He took us out of that back door again, and Bonnie again gasped at the view. An old well stood in the ground. He pointed to some figures on it. 'Look.' The numbers '1943' had been chiseled out of the stone. 'The year I was born,' he explained. 'My father did that to mark my arrival.' Then he gestured to the garden. 'Look, old fruit trees. Apples, pears, figs. You could plant more trees.' His arm swept across the land to the left. *'La piscine,'* he said smilingly, *'pour les enfants.'* He pointed towards the valley. *'Les montagnes.'* The Pyrenees. All I could see were clouds. When conditions are right, he said, you can see the peaks on the horizon. Bon visibly melted. How far? I asked. About an hour-and-a-quarter's drive south to the low slopes, he said, and an hour-and-a-quarter's drive east to the coast. I translated and Bon let out a satisfied sigh. Paradise, she said. Mountains and sea. Perfect.

With uncanny intuition, I was beginning to see the direction in which things were heading. But there was an obstacle, a bloody big overwhelming insurmountable ob-sta-cle. I had no money. How's that for a problem? Bon and I both had respectable incomes, but what with an eye-watering mortgage plus the amount I was paying in child support, we were far from living within our means. I had a world-class overdraft. I knew I couldn't afford a tent, let alone a rambling French farmhouse.

Jean-Pierre invited us back to his house to meet his wife. We sat in their *séjour*, along with the estate agent, sipping local wine and chatting. The small talk suddenly dipped and Jean-Pierre looked at me, raised his eyebrows, and said, *'Eh bien?'*

I stuttered and stammered, groping unsuccessfully for the French for 'mortgage' and 'overdraft'. He got a pencil and paper and scribbled some figures. He talked about the house, and the large piece of land to the left. 'They are for sale separately,' he explained, and pointed to the figures. The house: 250,000 francs, the land 60,000 francs. I did an easy calculation in my head, the French franc being then ten to the pound. £31,000. I shook my head, not in a clever negotiating kind of way, but a sort of *You don't understand, I am broke with a monstrous mortgage and overdraft* kind of way.

He immediately said, 'You don't have to buy the land, you can just buy the house, but I should point out there is planning permission on the land, so someone could build a house in what is in effect your garden.' I instantly shook my head. *Nobody is going to build a house in my bloody garden,* I thought.

I demurred again. It was simply not realistic, but the fact of the matter was my French was not good enough to explain to him the intricacies of my pathetic financial situation. So I said what I knew I could say. 'My wife and I would like to go back to our hotel and think about it.' Jean-Pierre and Claudette's faces fell so totally that Bonnie gasped. She whispered to me, 'We've made them so sad. It's awful.' I had to agree. What had these nice French people ever done to us that deserved us making them so sad?

Jean-Pierre looked at me with grief etched in his face. With barely audible voice, as if I was holding a red-hot poker to his chest, he said he could reduce the land by 10,000 francs. That's £30,000 I thought. It was, by any standards, amazing, a snip. A potentially beautiful old French farmhouse, with just the right amount of land, in the same family for generations, with the owner and his wife living just a few minutes away, the promise therefore of someone always to keep an eye out for us, look after it, and all in an area of France redolent with history. What a perfect contrast to Baker Street!

But I had no money. Minor problem. I tried once again to explain my financial situation, but I was embarrassed. I knew I was inviting the question 'Then why did you bother coming to look, if you can't afford to buy anything?' I struggled again, stuttering and stammering some more. This was not a ploy, not a clever piece of negotiating, it was a floundering struggle to explain in French that I did not have any money. Jean-Pierre clearly did not see it that way.

He took a deep breath, looked me in the eye, and said he would throw the land in. Free. For nothing. Everything for 250,000 francs, £25,000. There, he said. That is it. He gestured to his wife and the agent, and they got up and left the room.

Bon asked me what he had said. I stood up and paced for a few moments. I put my hands on her shoulders. 'He is offering us everything, the house and all the land, for £25,000.' 'Well, I don't think we can say no, can we?' Those were her exact words, and I can recall them precisely, 20 years less two months later.

It is August 2007 and my Admiral Nurse Ian has made a suggestion. 'Why don't you keep a journal?' he asked in one of our sessions. 'No,' I said, 'no time for that. Anyway, it wouldn't help. Why would it help? It'd just magnify everything, having to remember awful stuff and live through it again as I write it down.' 'I just thought that with you being a journalist, you are used to writing. You've written about that dead deaf hero of yours [Beethoven], you might find it helpful. You'd be able to refer back to it, which might help you deal with certain situations if they arise again.' 'No,' I said, 'definitely not.' I started writing that night.

I need a title, so I will call it 'Living with Dementia'. Bonnie doesn't know she has dementia. She knows she has begun to forget things, but she doesn't understand why. I know why, and that should make it easier for me to deal with. But for some reason it doesn't. She'll forget something, get something wrong, I'll get short with her, and she doesn't understand why.

That's why this journal is really more about me than her. I can see what's happening, so I get more upset than her. Ian said it would be a good idea for me to make a note if something goes wrong, then I'll know to handle it differently next time. That's what your next book should be, he said. It'll be helpful to you, and one day, maybe, helpful to other people who find themselves in a similar situation to you. I hesitated. It's all too personal. But really I knew that if I started, I wouldn't stop.

So I started. Here it is. A constant stream of words, written in the white heat of battle, as it were.

Now we had agreed to buy Tardan (the name the house has had for maybe 200 years, no meaning, just a name), I merely had to work out how to pay for it. Simple, really. For my entire adult life, I have worked on the principle that just because you can't afford something is no reason not to have it. I would open an account at Midland Bank in Paris and ask them for a mortgage, since interest rates in France were considerably lower than in the UK. Problem was, it would have to be a 100 per cent mortgage – I didn't have a bean to put towards it. Sounds familiar, I know, but the difference here was we were really not talking about a lot of money. In the lucky event the bank said *oui*, would I be able to afford the repayments? Of course not. It would just mean a larger overdraft, that was all. I was back on track at ITN, now a full-time newscaster with a very respectable salary (the BBC had tried to poach me for their new Breakfast show, which led ITN to upgrade my salary from respectable to very respectable), and Bonnie was working for Chuck and earning decently too.

Out of courtesy – and also hoping it would help to play the loyalty card – I went to see my local bank manager (the one and only Peter Thorne's successor), to ask her about opening an account with the sister bank in Paris. I explained about this wonderful property in France that I wanted to buy and for which I needed a mortgage. She thought for a moment and asked why I wanted the mortgage in France and not here, in London. I gave the obvious answer that interest rates in France were lower.

She frowned and pointed out that I would need to transfer money each month to my Paris account and the exchange rate could fluctuate, that it would cost me each month to make the transfer, and that who could tell, maybe interest rates in the UK would soon begin to come down. Then she said, 'Why don't you take out the mortgage here, from us? You won't have the exchange rate problem, and you won't have to pay charges each month to make the transfer. Plus it keeps everything very neatly together, right here.' I thought for a moment. 'But I already have a large mortgage with you, on our flat. Would you really be prepared to give me another one, at a hundred per cent, on a house in France?'

She smiled, sat back and folded her hands on her chest. 'Let me put it like this. We have absolutely no interest in your French farmhouse but we love your London flat, because given what has happened to property prices it's seriously under-mortgaged. So we could increase the mortgage on your flat, and you could use the money to buy the house in France.' For the second time in as many years, I wanted to kiss the manager of Midland Bank, Baker Street. (This one being female, it was considerably more tempting. No offence, Peter.)

Just as well I gallantly resisted the temptation, because within a very short time I wanted to strangle her. Interest rates in Britain continued to rise, and on a single notorious day in 1992 they hit 15 per cent. Our French farmhouse was crippling us.

It didn't last, of course, and over the years interest rates progressively fell. We had our house in France, and we kept it. We were living the dream. Dangerous talk.

✳ ✳ ✳ ✳

We are in Tardan. I was cooking dinner, punching way above my weight. I had decided to cook steaks – difficult for a good cook, impossible for me. I put them in the little oven that stands on the worktop (grilling would be too complicated for me because it would involve turning the steaks), opened the door every minute to check how things were going, and I reckoned they were just a few minutes off being ready. I was panicking, though. I was worried I hadn't got them right, and a storm was brewing up outside. That presented a problem. The large bedroom windows were open, and if the storm broke, water would come flooding in upstairs.

I told Bonnie I was worried about the storm, but I also needed to watch the steaks, to avoid overcooking them. 'Shall I go upstairs and close the bedroom windows?' she asked. 'Brilliant idea,' I said, 'but be quick.'

It was the last I saw of her for 10 minutes. The steaks were out and getting cold. I yelled upstairs. She finally came down, unable to grasp why I was so angry. I was more than angry. I was incandescent. I lost it. I shouted at her, screamed at her, swore at her. I don't need to put down the words, you can imagine. Just to think of what I said brings tears of guilt to my eyes. I kept it up for the best part of half an hour. She sat there, head down, looking sad, not fighting back. I realised, slowly, that she really didn't understand why I was so angry. Finally she pushed her plate away, said she didn't need to take all this abuse, and went upstairs. I took some deep breaths and calmed down. The full horror of what I had done sank in. Guilt is too weak a word.

I shall now go up and join her in bed. I hope she has forgotten about it and is asleep.

❋ ❋ ❋ ❋

'We are living the dream,' I said to Bon one evening, after a long drive down, sitting on the terrace drinking chilled rosé and watching the sun set over the valley.

Next morning, the shower water seemed to take longer than it should to run away. An hour later, Jean-Pierre and I were up to our knees in mud, digging up the garden and trying to fix the pipe leading to the septic tank.

There have been many of what I call my 'Greek island moments'. Like when I stood in the fireplace on a cold wet afternoon, struggling to remove the plaque across the bottom of the chimney. Finally – and suddenly – it came out, and I drowned in a sea of soot. *Why are we not on a Greek island?*

But the best (worst) of all, occurred seven years after we bought the house (yes, seven, you'll understand why). It was mid-August, and wet, very wet. Bon was cooking hot soup for lunch when the Butane gas cylinder ran out. No problem. Up into the dusty attic, unscrew the connecting pipe, lift the cylinder, down the rickety stairs, into the boot of the car, down the hill to Arlette, give her the empty, get a full one.

Back up into the attic, the full bottle weighing a ton, dump it on the dusty, mouse-dropping-ridden floor, treading carefully so as not to fall through suddenly to the kitchen, break the security seal on the cylinder, on my knees, screw the pipe back on … But it wouldn't go, it would not screw on. Try again. Wipe the sweat from my brow. Rain hammering on the roof and dropping through onto my hair. Knees sore from dirt and grit tearing through my jeans. The pipe would not screw onto the bottle.

OK, fine. Something wrong. Lug the bottle, still weighing a ton, down the stairs, into the back of the car, down the hill to Arlette, explain there is a problem, the pipe would not screw back on. Hmm, she looks puzzled, lifts her shoulders in a gesture of resignation, maybe there's something wrong with it, never mind, have another one. *Merci, merci, Arlette*. Back up the hill, up into the attic with the oh-so-heavy bottle, dump it on the floor, break the seal, on my knees, hurting now, screw the pipe back on, but it would not go, it bloody would not go on. Rain hammering on the roof and falling around me, knees seriously sore, and I have now woken the wasp nest in the eaves and there is buzzing ominously close to my head, sweat pouring.

Another dodgy bottle, back down the stairs, swing my arm back and half hurl it into the boot of the car, back down the slope. Arlette looks even more puzzled, strange that two should be not right, but never mind, *c'est la vie*, have another one, *bon courage, mon brave*. I thank her profusely again. Back up into the attic, rain still pouring down, wasps still buzzing, jeans torn and knees beginning to bleed, break the seal and would the sodding pipe screw on to the sodding bottle? It sodding well would not.

By now I was beyond caring. I was in a state of manic dysphasia (I made that up). I could barely speak or think coherently. Back out to the car with bottle number three, down the hill to Arlette, who took one look at me and, without saying a word, hastily gave me bottle number four and ran for cover.

Back up into the attic, and I am mumbling like a madman, cursing and swearing, dirt and sweat mingling on my brow, tears of frustration and anger coursing down my cheeks, inviting the wasps to sting me – bloody do it, I shouted at them, see if I care – drop to my knees and cry out loud with pain as dirt and grit and mouse droppings ingrain themselves in my broken skin, break the seal, and one last monumental effort, the pipe on to the bottle, and ... No, it would not go on. I fell to the dusty floorboards, a mess and a wreck. Defeated.

I appeared at the kitchen door, and Bon pulled out a chair for me. 'Sit down, calm down, it doesn't matter, don't worry.' I looked up at her and mumbled through tear- and dirt-stained eyes, 'Why are we not on a Greek island?'

I calmed down slowly, took a shower, washed my hair, put antiseptic cream on my knees, scrubbed at my hands until they were raw, and finally appeared half human. At the back of my mind, though, was the knowledge that we had no gas in the house. How would we cook dinner? Bon reassured me. There was one electric hob on the cooker, and she would use that.

Now it just happened that early that evening some neighbours, Jean-Maurice and Hélène, were due round for a drink, an *apéro*, as they say here. Bon sat me down before they arrived. 'Now be relaxed,' she said, 'please don't tell them all about your struggle with the gas. It's the last thing they'll want to hear about.' 'Absolutely, absolutely,' I said, 'don't worry, I won't say a word.'

They arrived, I poured a glass of wine, Bon put out some nibbles, and Jean-Maurice said, 'So, how are things, have you had a good afternoon?' 'Have I had a good afternoon?' I responded incredulously, '*have I had a good afternoon?* I'll tell you what sort of afternoon I have had.' Bon, although her French did not allow her to follow every word, could tell from my face and gestures that I was doing exactly what I had promised not to. She sighed resignedly. I related the sorry tale of the gas cylinders, and the fact that no fewer than four had been faulty in a row. Something wrong with the thread. Unbelievable, but true.

'But,' said Hélène in a calm soft voice, the accent of the south-west giving her French a beguiling charm, 'you know that the thread on Butane gas cylinders goes the other way? It's true. It is the only thing in the world where the thread goes anti-clockwise,' and she demonstrated with her fingers. '*Mais pourquoi?*' She shrugged and smiled.

I translated for Bon, my voice cracking with emotion. 'The thread goes the other way. Can you believe it? The sodding arseholic thread goes the other goddamned way.'

'*Oui,*' said Jean-Maurice, and he asked me if the bottle was still up in the attic. I nodded. '*Viens. Je te le montre.*' Up we went, up those same rickety stairs, into the dusty, dropping-ridden, damp from the rain, buzzing with wasps attic, where gas cylinder number four stood forlornly, its seal lying alongside it. He picked up the pipe, and gently screwed it onto the bottle, anti-clockwise. '*Voilà.*'

We came back down, and I have never enjoyed a glass of wine as much in my life.

The next morning, the phone rang. It was Arlette. 'I forgot to mention, did you know that the thread goes the other way?' I explained to her that Jean-Maurice had shown me, and that I was mortified, how could I ever apologise enough, and please, please, since I had broken the seal on three cylinders, may I please come back down and buy them all?

She laughed. 'How long did the original bottle last?' she asked. I did a swift calculation. 'Seven years.' She laughed again. 'That would mean you would have enough gas for twenty-one years. No, don't worry. I will give one to my brother, one to my uncle ...'

Ah yes, my Greek island moments. But our house, Tardan, has brought us incalculable pleasure down the years.

I have had a session with Ian. I told him about the steaks fiasco, and how I had lost it with Bon. I said I'd thought about it endlessly since, but didn't know how I could have done it differently.

He thought for a moment, then said, 'You watch the steaks, I'll run up and close the windows.'

So obvious, really, but it just never occurred to me. Emboldened, I said, 'Well, you can rest assured it will never happen again. I will never – never – lose my temper with her like that again.'

'Oh yes you will,' he said.

* * * *

At Philippe and Cathy's wedding 10 years or so ago, we met the real D'Artagnan. He drank more than anybody else, laughed harder than anybody else, sang louder than anyone else, danced more wildly than anyone else. I christened him the Chief Pisshead. He was Philippe's best man and he runs the local company that empties septic tanks. We belong to a small community in our village, people we have known for 20 years, and who have accepted us as their own. They have taught us about their way of life. And now they grieve with me for my Bonnie.

That dust-ridden attic is now a beautiful wood-panelled bedroom, probably the largest in south-west France. I am sitting writing this at our beautiful oak dining table, looking across at exactly where Bon and I sat that evening more than a decade ago, as Jean-Maurice and Hélène calmly explained about Butane threads. Bon is doing her walking. She sees me typing away, but asks no questions. I have a pit of nostalgia in my stomach.

How many times over the years have Bonnie and I gone through the story, repeated the mantra? *If* we had stayed at the hotel in the Pyrenees, *if* there had been a room at that hotel I telephoned on the coast, *if* there had been a room at any one of the hotels I went into in Capbreton, *if* we had stayed at the bed and breakfast, *if* we hadn't decided to have lunch in Aire, *if* we hadn't gone back to the agent's office after lunch … We would never have found Tardan.

I have never loved the English countryside, but down here in France it is different. Bonnie once explained to a friend in London that I had an aversion to English mud, but that somehow in France I didn't seem to mind. Why was this? The friend simply said, 'French mud'. There, that explains it perfectly.

Time for me now to bring the story full circle. I contacted Bob, and arranged for him and Sharon to come to our flat. They walked in, these two faces from our past. Bob, now in his early seventies, had lost his hair, but had the same wonderful Irish smile, and even more of a glint in his eyes. Easy to understand why. Sharon was as glamorous as ever, still dressed in white, sparkling, radiant, and now Bob's wife. (So Sharon joins Bonnie in proving once and for all – apologies, Bob – that there is hope for every man.)

Bob told us over dinner how he had lost his wife not so long ago, how Sharon's husband had left her for another man – we both shook our heads at the impossibility of that – how the two of them had got in touch, and how, yes, 19 years after Bob had failed to say '*Voulez-vous coucher avec moi?*', Sharon had finally said yes, and a lot more.

Bonnie sat with us, but it was obvious she had no memories of La Valouze or Bob and Sharon. Bob said to me later he had tried to engage her in conversation, but realised quickly that it was no use. But she seemed content, thank goodness.

So many memories, but none of them any longer shared.

Chapter 7

You'd think getting the diagnosis, being able to put a reason to things –
missing watch, missing passport, losing me at the airport, forgetfulness –
would turn me into an entirely understanding and forgiving husband to
the woman I adore. Sadly not.

One day in July 2007, we were preparing for a trip to France. It was
the most intense day of forelog I can remember. We were leaving the
next morning for a whole month. So much to get ready. I took the day
off work. I was in our flat, waiting for the mail, which I knew should
contain a rather large cheque. I was desperate to get it into the bank
before it closed. There had been a postal strike the day before. I laid
everything out: passports, euros, driving license. Also I had earmarked a
whole load of stuff from the fridge that needed packing. Still no mail
through the door. I had a lot of paperwork to get through, bills to pay.
Also loads of laundry to do. And at 4.30 I had an appointment with a
dermatologist for some minor surgery to remove a couple of growths on
my face.

I was running out of time. I phoned the porter to ask if the mail had
been delivered yet. Yes, but it's all in big sacks, unsorted. The bank would
close in an hour. I went down to the entrance hall. The porter must have
seen the look on my face. He opened sack after sack, went through what
seemed like hundreds of envelopes. Then I saw the letter I was waiting
for, and yes the cheque was inside.

I dashed to the bank, banged off a load of e-mails, finished the paperwork, got things ready for the morning because the damned flight was at

6.20am, which meant setting the alarm for 3.30, finished off the tumble drying, made sure we had dinner in – quick and easy, three minutes in the microwave – then left for the doctor. I was on an operating table, he gave me two local anaesthetics, one in my chin, the other in my cheek, which hurt like hell, and he gouged out the offending growths. I returned home looking like a war casualty, sticking plaster failing to hide the congealing blood underneath, waiting for the anaesthetic to wear off and the pain to kick in.

Deep down, I resented the fact I was having to do everything, absolutely everything. If things had been normal, Bon would have been doing all the domestic stuff while I concentrated on the 'manly' things. But I knew she could no longer do any of that. At last, I had it all done. Bank, paperwork, laundry, everything. I cooked dinner. We sat down. I had decided that with such an early start the next morning, we wouldn't have wine. Sod that. I opened a bottle, and the first glass went down without touching the sides of my throat.

I looked at Bon in triumph. I had done it. She smiled at me and said, 'Well done'. I took the steaming food out of the microwave and gave it to her to dish up. I sat down and smiled a satisfied smile. She reached forward for the salt cellar. She said, 'It's empty.' My head slumped forward onto my arms and the tears came.

* * * *

There was a cloud in my life: I hadn't seen my boys for around three years because of a series of court orders. I was forbidden to visit my eldest son at his boarding school in Oxford. My parents were not allowed to visit the two younger boys at boarding prep school, for fear they might kidnap them (no, really). In the first months after the divorce, the boys were allowed to come to my parents' flat (in the same block as ours, four floors below) but not up to our flat and not, absolutely not, allowed to see Bonnie (whom they remembered, of course, from the Henley years).

But coming to Mum and Dad's flat was soon stopped by another court order. All that was about to change.

Some time in late 1988 or it might have been early 1989, Bonnie said to me that I really ought to try to see my boys again, and I should apply to the courts to be allowed to do so. Frankly I blanched at the prospect of more meetings with lawyers, more legal letters, more costs that we could not afford.

I confided to a senior ITN reporter, female, that my total happiness at living with Bonnie was clouded by just one thing. I was not seeing my boys. She said, 'Don't worry. One day they will want to see you, and they will put things right themselves.' I told her I thought she was wrong. 'You'll see,' she said.

There I was one afternoon, sitting in the small Superchannel newsroom at the top of the building, when the telephone alongside me rang. It was Mary in reception. 'Hi, John. Your son is here to see you.'

Outwardly I stayed calm; inside my nerve ends jangled, my stomach somersaulted, my throat tightened, my eyes moistened. I was able to suppress any sound, so no heads turned. All I could think to say was 'Which one?' 'Which one are you?' I heard Mary ask. A young man's voice, which I didn't recognize, answered 'Damian'. 'Damian,' said Mary. 'Thanks, I'll be right down.'

I got up and walked to the lift, breathing shallowly. What did this mean? Why had he come? Was he angry with me? In the lift I prepared myself for the worst. I walked to reception feeling like a condemned man walking to his fate. Whatever the reason, I had been an absent father, so I deserved whatever I was about to get. The small reception area was quite full. I swept my eyes round the seats, but couldn't see my son. I swept my eyes round again, and noticed a young man I didn't recognise, with long hair and a stubbly face, pointing at himself.

He stood, walked towards me, gestured to the entrance, we walked outside, and he threw his arms round me. We hugged and sobbed.

People came up the steps into the building, out of the doors and down the steps. We didn't care. We just hugged and sobbed.

Finally we separated. I looked at him. The boy had become a young man. We talked, breathlessly. He said Kieran and Rory both knew he had come, but no one else knew. He said, 'Dad, we want to see you, all of us, we really want to see you.' Then he said he had to go. We had a last quick hug, and he ran down the steps and away.

❊ ❊ ❊ ❊

And so I braced myself and set the legal ball rolling. I got a result, of a kind. I was to be allowed to see my children, but only if I went to the old family home in Henley, took them out for a maximum of four hours, and promised in writing that I would be alone (in other words, not with Bonnie) and that I wouldn't attempt to take them to London, to my flat or my parents' flat, or anywhere outside the environs of south Oxfordshire.

The law is a [*sic*] ass, wrote Charles Dickens in *Oliver Twist*. No, really, Mr Dickens, whatever gave you such a foolish notion? I prefer an expression we used to use regularly in the newsroom – LJS, or Loony Judge Syndrome.

So I began to see my boys again, to experience that awkward curse of divorce, the lone parent attempting to amuse the children during a short period of access. On the second or third such visit, I took them to lunch in Reading, then we went for an hour to a newly opened dry ski slope. I was wearing a new grey leather jacket, which Bon had bought me. On my second or third downhill run, I had a spectacular wipe-out, tearing my knees, elbows and the jacket. The boys laughed like drains, and whatever the motive it was so good to see them doubled up with laughter that I joined in happily.

It was a curious kind of limbo between not seeing the boys at all and leading a normal life, and I couldn't see how I could ever progress to normality. Little did I know it, but I was about to achieve just that. My ex-wife, an experienced teacher, had for some years wanted to return to the US, and in 1989 she landed a job at a school close to Washington DC. She planned to accept the job and take the two younger boys to the US with her.

I received a letter to this effect from her solicitor. It stated my ex-wife's intention, adding that this would mean a variance of the court order, which would require my signature. The necessary papers would be forwarded to me shortly. Another bloody lawyer's letter. Was it going to begin again? Hadn't we left all that behind?

Then I received a piece of legal advice that changed everything. Basically, I was in a good bargaining position. If my ex-wife wanted me to agree to my sons living in the States, she would have to give me full and free access to them. That's what happened and soon I was seeing my children again, this time without ridiculous restrictions. They would be able to come back to the UK for holidays, they could come to my flat while Bonnie was there, and they could see their grandparents. Normal life could be resumed, with work on my part. The boys had been hurt, badly, and I knew I had to shoulder my share of the blame for that. But if the courts had exercised just a tiny bit more humanity, a lot of it could have been avoided.

My children are now adults, with children of their own. They have worked through their hurt, and understand why things happened as they did. And what of my relations with them now? I recently met a retired schoolmaster and asked him what he did, how he kept himself busy. 'I am banker and chauffeur to my kids,' he said. Ah yes, the bliss of parenthood, grandparenthood, retirement. That's not a complaint. I wouldn't have it any other way.

✳ ✳ ✳ ✳

No more breakdowns. I absolutely swore no more breakdowns. This morning I had a breakdown. We're in our French farmhouse. Bon's brother Bill and his wife, who live in San Francisco, are arriving tonight for a couple of days. Make up their beds, put out towels, sweep upstairs, clean the bath, decide meals, make a food shopping list. In the shower, I realised we needed a new bar of soap. That set me off.

'Could you sweep upstairs while I do the food list?' 'Yes, but I don't know where the brooms are.' 'They're where they've always been.' For years she has kept a Pliz broom and wipes in the corner of our bedroom. She always claimed it was therapeutic moving the French broom, with the silly name and the soft wipes that clip to its base, slowly and gently across the parquet floor.

We went shopping and I was cruel to her. Come on, keep up, even though I knew her hip was hurting. What really gets to me is that she doesn't make decisions any more. What shall we get? Some of that, she'll say, pointing at the nearest thing. No idea. Absolutely no idea. In the car going home, I was still having a go about her doing nothing any more. I do it all. Everything. 'Do you know what I did this morning? Everything. Every fucking thing. You don't even Pliz any more.' 'I don't know where the Pliz is – I looked for it but couldn't find it.'

That's when I realised she wasn't being difficult, not being awkward. She really didn't know where the Pliz was, where it's been for years gone by. The tears welled up in my eyes and my throat tightened.

So this morning, by having a breakdown, I broke my own rule, the lesson I have learned from Ian. When I have a breakdown, the only person who suffers is me. She suffers, of course, but only because of what I inflict on her. And she can't do anything to make it better. That's the point. I keep fighting it, wanting her to fly in the face of it. But she can't.

I said earlier I would be reporting from the white heat of battle. Now I realise how wrong that is. This isn't a battle. There's no fighting it. It's not like cancer. You can't defeat it. You just have to go along with it. It can only get worse. It is beyond words cruel.

* * * *

In November 1991 my mum was admitted to hospital and it became clear to us all that she wasn't going to get better. When the senior physician took us to one side in February or March to tell us he didn't think Mum would be leaving hospital, it came as no surprise.

Dad, retired surgeon, was in his element, back in a hospital. I remember his quiet shock as the young houseman came to shake his hand in the ward, wearing a sloppy sweater and jeans. He redeemed himself by calling Dad 'Sir'. 'In my day,' Dad explained later, 'it was always a white coat, and the length of it denoted seniority.'

Mum's condition continued to deteriorate. In April, things took a turn for the worse. I took some time off. She died in May, and I miss her more now, all these years later, than ever.

Dad was a lost soul after she died. He was several years older than Mum, and it wasn't meant to be this way. I remember Mum laughing and joking about how, after Dad went, she and her best friend Peggy would go round the world having fun. Dad was a pretty serious man – I suppose it comes with his job. Mum was always game for a laugh – comes from being daughter of a photojournalist, I suppose. She used to call Dad a miserable old sod, and most of the time he was. When we were small, I remember Mum tickling him in the ribs to try to get a laugh from him. 'Stop it, Joan, stop it,' he would say quite angrily, the smile never coming to his face.

Well, it didn't happen the way Mum intended. The Top Man had other ideas, and she went first. My brothers and I moved Dad out of the large flat they had lived in on the second floor of Chiltern Court, and into a smaller one on the same floor as Bon and me. It meant I could keep an eye on him. Mostly his days consisted of sitting in an armchair with a couple of newspapers, and watching television in the evening. He took to cooking rice, and this he did most nights – only ever boiled, but it kept him busy. Occasionally Bon would cook an extra portion of our dinner and I would walk it round to him, or sometimes he would join us. Bon tried to persuade him to come and live with us, but he wouldn't even countenance the idea.

It was sad to see the extent to which he gave up. Here was a man, born in 1908 in South Africa, who had worked his way to England as a ship's doctor, qualified in medicine in London, and become one of the foremost surgeons of his generation. He had worked with Alexander Fleming on penicillin ('a good lab technician, that's all Fleming ever was,' Dad used to say dismissively), he pioneered painless childbirth and he improved the technique of hysterectomy to such an extent that he used to have the patient up and walking within days as opposed to weeks. When the BBC made a series in the late 1980s about how birth control had transformed women's lives, they beat a path to Dad's door. But after retirement he lost interest in all things medical.

Occasionally an old story would come out. 'This whole area around Baker Street was a red-light district during the war,' he said, 'and what nationality of soldier do you think had the highest incidence of syphilis?' 'American,' I replied confidently. 'Close. Canadian.' 'Why Canadian?' He shrugged his shoulders.

'Dad, you've got so many stories to tell,' I used to say to him, 'you don't have to write them down, just tell them to me and I'll write them.' But no, he wouldn't.

One day, a couple of years after Mum died, Bonnie had a brilliant idea, a brainwave. 'Why don't you encourage him to go back to visit South Africa?' she said. 'He'd never go,' I replied. 'He might. Why not suggest it? See what he says.' 'I'm telling you, he'd never go.' 'Why don't you take him?' I gulped.

I've just got to be more positive. Monsieur Negative, that's me. Always seeing the worst side of everything. Last night, down here in France, sister-in-law Denise cooked us supper. As soon as she started, Bon joined in. There she was, cutting up vegetables, enjoying it. She hasn't done that for ages.

What this means is that if I can just stop being negative, and see the positive in each situation, she'll be much better. I've got to learn to cook, start enjoying it, and it'll ignite a spark in her to do it as well. She used to be a fabulous cook – she just needs re-inspiring. Maybe, if I try hard enough, I could persuade her to knock up one of her world-famous trifles.

Denise and I had a long conversation on the terrace in the afternoon. I was negative, negative, negative. I've lost my Bonnie. I no longer live with the same person I fell in love with and adored. Denise nodded, which rather upset me. I hoped she would tell me it wasn't true. At least then we had the kitchen scenes, which made things a little better.

We've just remade the guest beds for the next guests coming down tomorrow, my son's in-laws. I had to sort out which new sheets, pillow-cases to put on, strip the beds and get the old stuff washed. She just looked on, tried to help with the beds, but there I was organising everything. I've asked her to sweep up insects and fluff from the floors upstairs. I gave her the famous Pliz mop and dustpan and brush, and she's doing it. Now I've got to think about food for the next few days. Oh yes, there's laundry (our bedclothes) to fetch from the dry cleaners in the nearest town about 10 miles away. I'll have to fit that in somehow.

My head is bursting. I need a cup of lemon tea. I go into the kitchen, snatch the serrated knife from the rack, slam it onto the lemon, and slice through my thumb.

The in-laws' visit went very well. I won't list all the small lapses of memory Bon had, the difficulties when she misunderstood something. I'm being positive. It really went well. We've now got a day-and-a-half before my son and his wife come down. I'm determined not to have a repeat of the last catastrophic in-between-guests breakdown.

I almost lost it twice this morning, after planning the meals, doing a long shopping list, doing the shopping, starting the washes going, and so on, when I found I had put the melons on top of the plums in the basket, squashing them, and the *croque monsieurs* I did in the oven came out with the tin foil sticking to the bottom of them. Minor, and I got over it.

I'm not rushing at it this time, but doing it at a leisurely pace. I was washing up after lunch and Bon was about to go up for her rest when she said, 'Thank you for doing the washing up.' I muttered, 'And the shopping, cooking, cleaning …', then stopped myself. It made me realise how bitter I could let this thing get. I smiled and said, 'You're welcome.' Result.

✳ ✳ ✳ ✳

I sat with Dad one evening in his flat and turned the conversation gently round to South Africa. I mentioned his brother's widow, talked about their children, my cousins. He smiled, enjoying the conversation. I talked particularly about my cousin Natalie, and how we had played together as children in the shadow of Table Mountain. That allowed me to bring up the family trip to Cape Town in 1947, yes, all those years ago, when I was three and brother David just one. He nodded, smiling nostalgically at the memory. I talked about standing on a lighted cigarette end on the deck of the *Windsor Castle*, and if I think hard enough can still almost feel the pain. I told him I resented the fact that when I accidentally sent my new clockwork car over the side, he refused to ask the captain to stop the ship and send a diver down to retrieve it.

I always thought that had just been a family trip for Dad to show off his English wife and children to his parents and relatives, but I found out much later that he had actually considered moving us all there, in which case my brothers and I would have been brought up under apartheid. The only reason he didn't was because Dad's strictly Jewish mother wouldn't accept my non-Jewish grandmother as one of the family. So

Dad said, 'Well, if that's your attitude, you can all go and play marbles' –
classic Dad expression – and he brought us back to London. How different our lives might have been!

I chose my moment and said, 'You know what, Dad? Why not take a
little trip back to Cape Town? See the family. Your old haunts. What do
you say?' The smile left his face instantly. 'Don't be silly. I can't.
Impossible.' I paused, then said, 'Do you remember how long it took you
to go back when Granddad died? Two days, or thereabouts, and –' He
picked up the oft-told story, 'I had to go by flying boat across the
Mediterranean, then another small plane across Africa. It took at least
two days.' I smiled. 'Overnight, now. That's all. Get on the silver bird at
Heathrow, go to sleep, wake up, and you're there.'

A small smile played on his lips, but he said nothing. I continued in the
same vein. 'Do you remember, when we were kids, how you used to
phone the family in Cape Town every Christmas? You used to have to
book the call with the operator, then we would all gather round the phone
24 hours later, it would ring on cue, and we used to speak to those crackly
voices way down there near the Antarctic.' He liked that, more smiles.
'Things have changed so much, and it's all down to communications,' I
said, 'as you have so often reminded me. Now, we just pick up the phone,
and – boof! – we are speaking instantly to Cape Town. Same with travel.
No more flying boats. Leave tonight, you're there for breakfast, and in
comfort too. What about it, Dad? Why not? It would be wonderful, so
many memories, and so easy to do. And just imagine how pleased they'd
be to see you. Lee, your brother Harry's wife, you haven't seen her for
decades. And the girls, Natalie and Hazel, and their children.' 'Don't be
silly,' he said, 'I couldn't do it. I'm 86 years of age. You've got to be young
to fly all the way down there.' I paused, to let his words hang in the air.
'You could do it, you know, and what's more it would take years off you.'
'I couldn't do it alone,' he shot back, 'you know that.'

He had walked right into my carefully laid trap. 'Tell you what. Let
me take you. I'm owed a bit of holiday by ITN. What do you say?' He

looked at me in a state of shock. He knew I had outgunned him, and he was secretly thrilled to his boots. He continued to look at me, eyes wide, mouth open. I shot out of the chair. 'Don't say a thing. Leave it to me. Guess what? I'm taking you back to Cape Town.'

* * * *

By September 2007, I was beginning to worry about leaving Bon on her own during the day while I was at work. Her cousin Carol came over from the US again and told me she too was worried. She felt Bon needed a companion, someone to talk to, someone to make sure everything was ok. I stalled for a while – I can cope, can't I? But her words weighed on me. One evening at dinner, I asked Bon what she had done while I was at work. She looked confused and shook her head. That was a worry. If she couldn't remember what she had done that afternoon, who could tell what she might do and not remember? I decided to take action.

My Polish daughter-in-law, Dorota, Kieran's wife, told me to leave it to her. She put an ad on a website that she knew was a favourite with Poles in the UK. It said simply that a housekeeper/carer was required for a professional couple in central London, and that the successful applicant should be prepared to go down to France with them as required. She received more than 200 replies, whittled them down to a shortlist of 30, whittled that down to two, and highlighted the one she thought was perfect for the job. I disagreed. The other of the two had worked for the elderly mother of a Roman Catholic priest. Perfect. Dorota told me to interview them both. I did. Dorota was right. Monika was the one.

I remember opening to the door to a smiling young Polish woman. Bon and I sat opposite her on either side of the dining table. She was relaxed, calm, positive, rarely stopped smiling. Even when I told her I wanted her to take care of all the meals, and she expressed slight concern about not knowing what we liked to eat, the smile stayed put. I tried to see through it – all those articles on how to behave in interviews say to keep smiling and appear confident – but it really did seem genuine. We even digressed a little and talked about history. I can't remember how a medieval Polish king entered the conversation, but I found myself recounting one of my favourite legends: how, when the Turkish army reached the gates of Vienna in 1683, it was largely thanks to a Turkish-speaking Polish double agent, who sneaked out of the besieged city into the Turkish camp and beyond to raise the alarm, and that King Sobieski of Poland rode to the rescue, and the Turks left behind coffee beans, which the double agent used to open the first café in Vienna … Yes, your eyes have glazed over, but Monika's didn't. She even told me that a village right next to her home town was named after Sobieski, and she had been born there. Well, she'd got the job before she left the flat.

At no point during this process – the ad, the replies, the interviews – did Bonnie ever ask me why we were doing this, why we needed someone to come in and cook and clean for us. She simply accepted that if I had decided this was what we needed, then this was what we needed. A couple of times I said something to the effect that Mum and Dad always had a housekeeper, and that it took so much strain off them, and here we were doing the same thing, and it would make life a lot easier for us, we wouldn't have to worry about this or that. But I needn't have said a word. Bonnie never questioned anything.

There was more to my cunning plan. An idea had been forming in my mind, but I had not let myself think about it until I cleared the first hurdle, namely getting Dad to agree (or not disagree) about letting me take him to South Africa. That hurdle cleared, I moved on to Phase Two.

'Isn't it amazing news about Dad agreeing to the South Africa trip?' I said to Bonnie one evening in the kitchen, as I handed her a glass of wine. 'You were right. Me offering to take him was the clincher. Cheers.

Here's to the trip.' Dramatic pause. Then, 'Love, look, why don't you come with us?'

'No. Your dad wouldn't want me to come. It's just you and him. It'll be good for you both.'

I was taken aback. I was prepared for her to say she was too busy at work and wouldn't be able to get time off, or that something was happening at home she couldn't miss, but Dad not wanting her to come was a line I'd never thought of, and I knew immediately she was wrong. 'Of course he wouldn't want you not to come,' I said, muddling my words. 'He would love you to come, honestly, I know he would. He would love it.' 'No,' she said with finality, 'he wouldn't, and I forbid you to ask him.'

I raised it a couple of times in the ensuing few days, but always got the same response. I hadn't yet done anything about planning the trip. I knew I had to look at flights, and also telephone cousin Natalie to talk things through – when would be a good time, where should we stay, could she book somewhere, and so on? But the more I thought about it, the more I wanted Bonnie to come. I knew instinctively Dad wouldn't mind, and I wanted so much for her to meet the Cape Town branch of the family. I thought about asking Dad, then telling Bon the good news, but I didn't want to go behind her back. So I tried one more time. 'Let me ask him.' That was all I said. She surrendered gracefully.

'Dad,' I said that evening in his flat. 'I'm about to plan everything for Cape Town. How would you feel if Bonnie came with us?' Honestly, my memory has not embellished his reaction with the passage of time. 'Rather,' he said (a favourite affirmative of his), saying it in about four or five syllables, his eyes opening wide and twinkling with pleasure. I smiled quietly and said I would arrange it.

I had no problem changing Bonnie's mind for her. I told her Dad's reaction, put my arms round her, and said, 'You're coming.'

Natalie screamed with delight when I phoned her, insisted that Dad would stay with his sister-in-law Lee (her mother) and that Bon and I would stay with her and her husband ('we have an entire basement flat').

And so, in early December 1994, Bonnie and I boarded a British Airways flight to take my Dad back to his roots.

Monika is superb. She knows about Bonnie's diagnosis, of course, and it hasn't fazed her one bit. She seems to know exactly how to behave with Bon. She has been a carer before, for very elderly and infirm women. At the moment she doesn't need to do a lot regarding Bonnie's care, but she understands that things will, in time, take their course. For now, she is housekeeper first, carer second.

Monika plans meals the day before, makes shopping lists, does the cooking. Bon has not eaten so much and as well for a long time. Of everything, this whole food issue is probably the biggest weight off my shoulders. And Monika actually enjoys it! Thinking of ways to do this and that, making it different. She added hard-boiled eggs to a salad yesterday. When I have bought eggs, I haven't thought of any other way of using them except as boiled eggs at breakfast. Same with ham. I always buy ham, then put it on a plate for lunch. Monika cuts it up and adds it to a creamy pasta. Who would have thought of it? I have just heard her announce she is going to wipe out the fridge. She is a miracle worker!

It was a magical week. I photographed Dad as he stepped off the aircraft steps on to South African soil, this frail elderly man who had first left his country more than 60 years before.

Natalie and I hugged and laughed and joked and remembered. Dad, always so reluctant to show his emotions, put his arms round his brother's widow and hugged her more than I had ever seen him hug anyone before. The family welcomed my Bonnie with open arms. On the Friday evening at dinner, they prepared for the weekly Jewish ritual and all that muttering and religious mumbo jumbo that makes my skin crawl. I stepped back from the table and said, You'll have to excuse me, I can't do this. They understood, and instead of berating me (which they were perfectly entitled to do), they laughed at my cynicism. Bonnie, on the other hand, took my breath away by going over to Lee and saying, 'Explain it to me. I want to know about it. It seems a lovely tradition.' Lee's face was a picture, and the look she shot at me was not one of 'There, see?' but 'You are truly lucky to have such a wonderful wife'.

As for Dad, well, with Lee driving and navigating, we visited every house he had lived in for the first two decades of his life. Not only was each and every one still there, but Dad remembered them all, giving us the addresses and setting each one in its place in his memory. We visited the house he had lived in when just a toddler, and opposite it was the mound of concrete that was a memorial to some family members who had died in the nineteenth century and were buried underneath. 'I used to climb on that when I was a child,' he said.

At the next house he fell silent, standing in the middle of the street looking up. I left him alone for a few moments with his memory, then went up to him. Softly he said, 'Do you see that white balcony there, on the first floor?' and he pointed up to it. 'I used to sit on that balcony with my dad, and he taught me so much. There. Just there. On that balcony.' He fell silent again, and his eyes misted over. I calculated that this must have happened more than 70 years before.

One excursion took us to the beautiful wine town of Franschhoek, about an hour's drive from Cape Town. Dad told us that as a student, trying to earn enough money to get to England, he had worked in the café at the local train station. I took a photograph of Bonnie and Dad in Franschhoek, and it is one of my very favourite photos. Dad, elderly, frail, his face earnest but content in a way I had rarely seen before, and Bonnie, utterly beautiful, a radiant smile on her face, and her arm protectively round my dad. It brings tears to my eyes just thinking of it, never mind looking at it.

We left with hugs and kisses, vowing to repeat the trip, but of course knowing we wouldn't. Bonnie said, 'You have come to know your Dad in a way you never would have if he had gone before your mum.' It was a wise comment. My memory now of my Dad is of how he was on that trip to South Africa, not of the rather distant, serious figure I had grown up with.

Within a year, Dad went into serious decline. He began to leave the hot tap in the kitchen running, and was unsure how to turn on the electric rings on the cooker. My brothers and I made the heart-rending decision that he needed full-time care in a care home. He resisted to the end. The night before Bonnie and I were due to take him, he said he would never go, never, never, never. The next morning when I went round to his flat at eight o'clock in the morning, he had his overcoat and hat on and was sitting on his suitcase in the hallway.

Bonnie and I drove him out to the home we had selected in Hertfordshire. Arm in arm, we walked him round the garden, then accompanied him to his room. Taking leave of him was one of those moments you don't forget. Bon squeezed my arm. We sat in the car and I had a cry. We both agreed he'd be out within a fortnight – he simply wouldn't accept it. In the event, he was there for four years.

I made a small photo album of the South Africa trip, all the houses he had known as a child, and leafed through it with him time after time on countless visits, and always he could give me the addresses. He languished in the home, in steady decline, before, at the age of 93, joining Mum at last. In fact, he should have done that on our return from South Africa. It was the perfect time, before his decline which caused him such grief – 'I'm a doctor, I know what is happening to me … Forgive me, I know I am talking rubbish … I'm going slowly bonkers, I'm sorry … Where's Mum, has she gone?' – and all of us such distress.

Lee, too, died soon after the visit. I didn't tell Dad. Most tragically of all, my lovely cousin Natalie, three weeks older than me and with whom I had frolicked as a toddler, died in 2008 of cancer. And you tell me there is a God?

* * * *

Bon has taken to carrying her house keys around the flat on a small tray, along with sunglasses, mobile phone and several glasses of water. Yesterday I saw her credit card wallet on the tray, which was on the surface immediately above the small drawer where I make sure all her important stuff is – wallet, credit cards, travel card, passport and so on. Occasionally one or more items will go missing. I usually find it in a handbag or coat pocket. The travel card vanished around nine months ago and has never turned up.

She was standing by the tray, so I said, 'Why don't I put your credit card wallet in the drawer?' She looked confused, and a little angry. 'Why?' 'Well, that way we'll know where it is. Shall I do it?' I reached forward. She stopped me. 'I'll do it,' she said, picked up the credit card wallet … and put it back down on the tray. 'Great,' I said, 'but why don't I put it in the drawer?'

She shook her head, had no idea what I was talking about, and headed for the door. As she passed me, she said in an exasperated voice, 'Bonnie at confused dot com'.

I laughed out loud, uproariously, spontaneously. It was a truly hilarious comment. I laughed on and on, doubled up. 'Well, it's true,' she said, smiling.

I think it was the biggest and best laugh I have had for two years – certainly since this nightmare started.

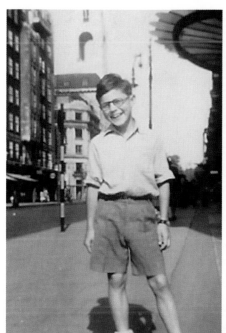

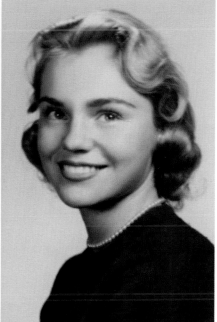

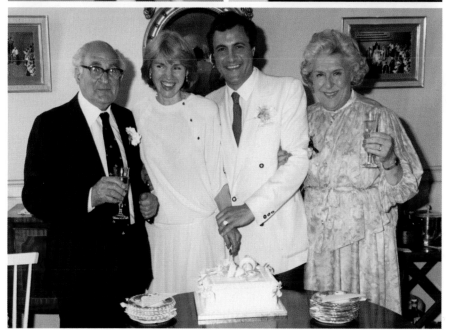

Top Left: Me outside Chiltern Court, c.1956.
Top Right: Bonnie, aged 19, soon to be Cornell Homecoming Queen.
Bottom: With Mum and Dad on our wedding day, 29th June 1985.

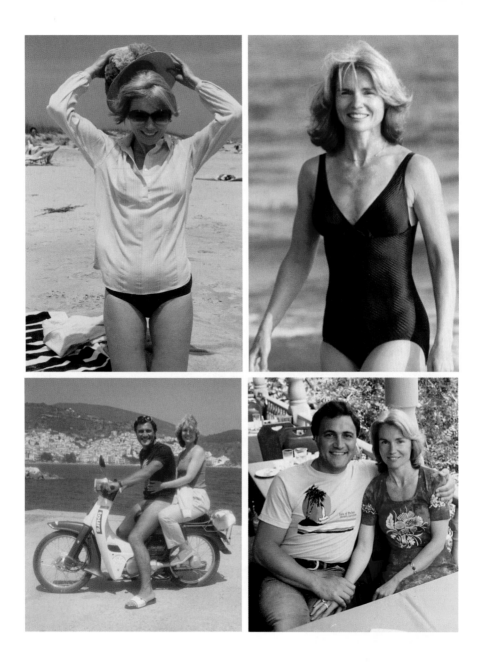

Top Left: Isle of Palms, South Carolina, wearing her mum's straw hat.
Top Right: Newport, Rhode Island: a favourite picture.
Bottom Left: Belated honeymoon on Skopelos, May 1986.
Bottom Right: Lunch in Charleston, South Carolina, photo by a Dutch tourist.

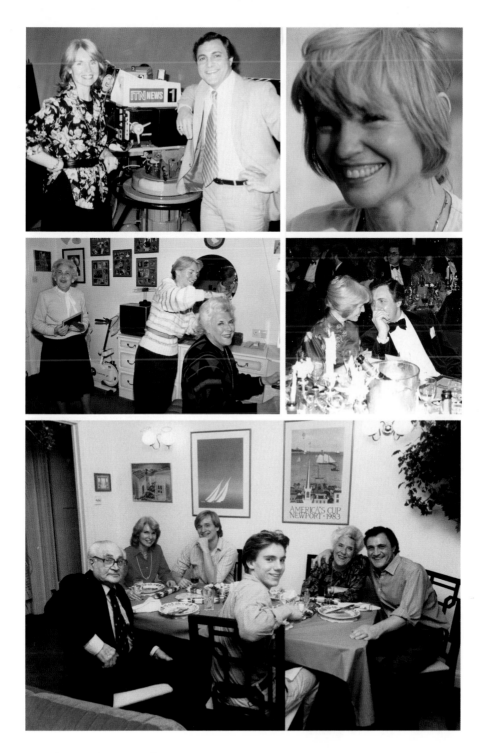

Top Left: The reporter becomes a newscaster.
Top Right: She really did find my jokes funny.
Middle Left: Bonnie gives my mum a trendy hairdo, with my aunt looking on.
Middle Right: A private moment before I accepted an RTS award for my Philippines coverage, February 1987.
Bottom: Dinner in our flat with Mum and Dad, and Bon's sons Alec (next to her) and H.

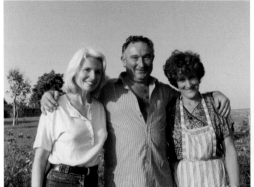

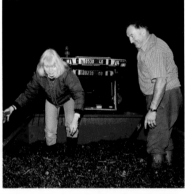

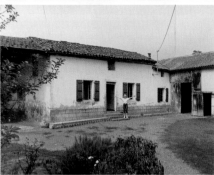

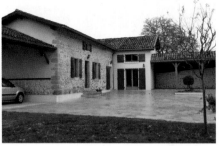

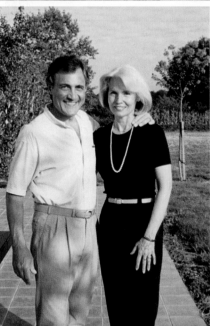

Top Left: Bonnie with Jean-Pierre and Claudette, on the day we found Tardan, August 1989.

Top Right: Helping Jean-Pierre with the grape harvest.

Middle Left: Tardan before (1989) …

Middle Right: … and after (2003).

Bottom: On the back terrace at Tardan.

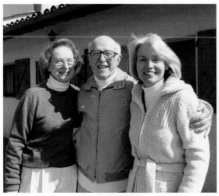
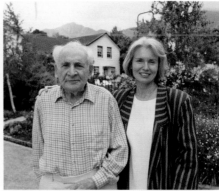
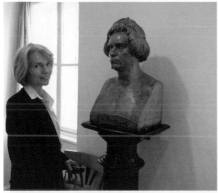
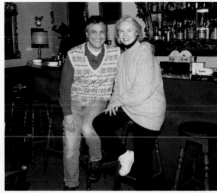
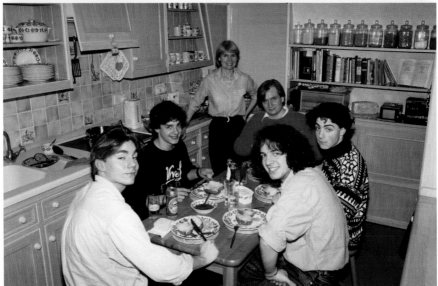

Top Left: Bonnie with her dad and stepmum at Tardan.
Top Right: Bonnie with my dad in Franschhoek, South Africa, an all-time favourite picture.
Middle Left: Keeping a straight face in front of the Master.
Middle Right: In the *Zum Alten Blumenstock*, Vienna, one of Beethoven's favourite haunts.
Bottom: All five boys together at last in our flat, December 1990.

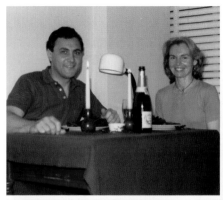

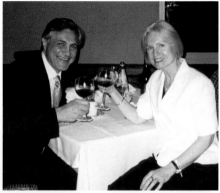

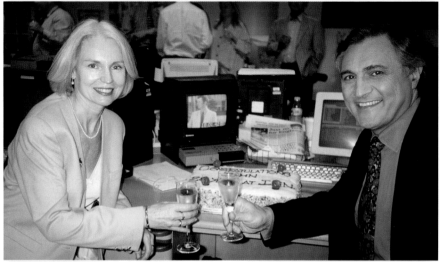

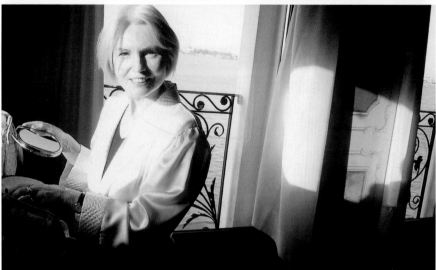

Top Left: The first dinner, Washington DC, 27th April 1983.
Top Right: The 20th anniversary dinner, Venice.
Middle: Celebrating 25 years at ITN, August 1997.
Bottom: 'Do you want me to be on time or not?' Preparing for the Venice anniversary dinner.

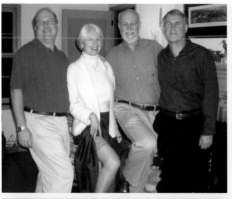
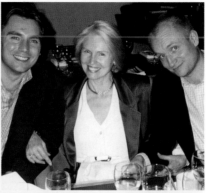
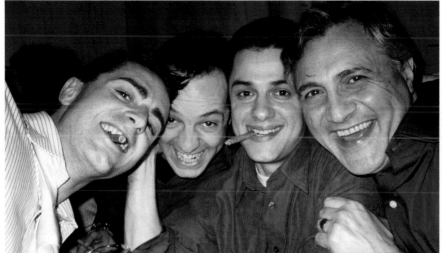
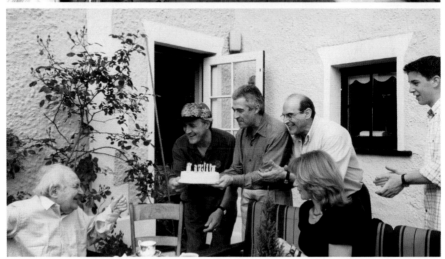

Top Left: Proving she's better looking than her brothers, Jon, Bob and Bill.
Top Right: With her sons H and Alec on her 60th birthday, 8th June 2001.
Middle: With my sons Rory, Damian and Kieran, at Damian's 30th birthday party,
February 2001.
Bottom: Brothers Peter, David and I present Dad with his cake on his 90th birthday,
May 1998.

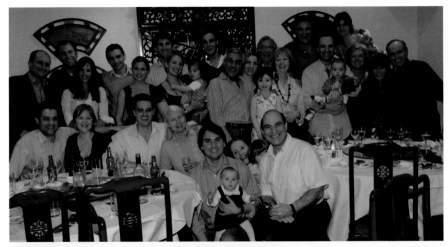

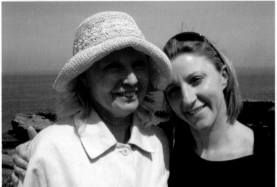

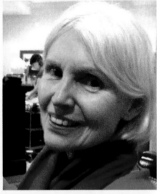

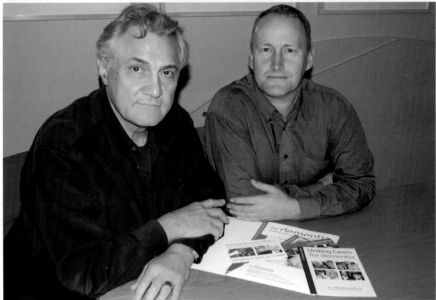

Top: Three generations of our families, April 2008.
Middle Left: Bonnie with the wonderful Monika.
Middle Right: Resident in Sundial, and still smiling.
Bottom: With my Admiral Nurse, Ian Weatherhead, after 'going public' about Bonnie's dementia, the strain clearly showing.

Chapter 8

Somewhere around 1993 or thereabouts, a third person entered our marriage. But Bonnie had nothing to worry about. First he was male, he was long dead, and anyway deaf as a post. Yes, Van the Man. Why Beethoven? What is it about his music that, for me, no other composer can match? It inspires me, lifts my spirit, encourages me, drives me, reinforces my belief in myself, yet also soothes and comforts me. Whatever my mood, there is something of his to reach for. The knowledge that he suffered the worst fate that can befall a musician – deafness – yet overcame it, inspires me all the more.

The idea of writing about Beethoven was like a seed that took root and flowered. A pretty slow-growing one, though. It was in 1983 that Bonnie first urged me to write his story, and a decade later when I typed the first words. The image that sparked it off was a passage in a dense biography describing how, at the age of 10, the boy Ludwig had sat with his mother on the deck of a boat taking them to Holland, where he was to play piano for the wealthy. It was so bitterly cold on board that he sat with his feet in his mother's lap, and she was rubbing them to stop them getting frostbitten.

This was about as far removed from the image we have of this godlike creature, laurel leaves around his head, wild hair flowing, eyes shooting out shards of intensity, lips downturned with determination and defiance, as it was possible to imagine. He was, after all, a boy who became a man, a human being with all the failings of humanity. A genius, yes, but that didn't stop his feet getting cold.

Bracing myself, I went to my ancient typewriter. What I wrote was brilliant – so brilliant that it disappeared in the first rewrite, never to reappear. But I had begun the first of thousands upon thousands of words I would write about this man. Five books published so far, a sixth under way, and I know what the seventh will be. Obsessed? Passionate is a better word.

＊　＊　＊　＊

This morning, Bon came in to breakfast dressed. Always she is in a dressing gown, then showers after breakfast. I pointed it out, she laughed and said she'd shower after breakfast and didn't know why she had got dressed first.

After breakfast, she showered. She then told me she would shower. I laughed and told her that she'd be really clean if she showered again. She laughed and said she meant she'd get dressed. I said phew. Into the bathroom she went and showered again.

Fuck, fuck, fuck, fuck, fuck.

＊　＊　＊　＊

'I think we need to go to Vienna for a long weekend,' I said at breakfast one Saturday morning in 1994. 'Yes, that should do it. I think I can do all the research I need in a long weekend.' I was just slightly out. In the end we went to Vienna three times (it may have been four), Prague twice, Bohemia north and south, central and lower Austria … In fact, we went to every place that Beethoven ever went that is still there to be seen. We walked and walked and walked. We talked late into the night, night after night.

There is one great mystery in Beethoven's life. Who was the woman to whom he wrote a passionate love letter, which he almost certainly did not send, but which he kept hidden in a drawer of his desk for the rest of his life? In that long letter, written in three parts, he calls her *meine unsterbliche Geliebte* (my immortal beloved), but he does not use her name once, as if he dared not risk it becoming known. But from other details he includes, the woman in question has to have been well known to Beethoven in Vienna, she has to have been in Prague in the first week of July 1812, where their brief love affair took place, and in the Bohemian spa town of Karlsbad in the weeks following, while Beethoven was in another Bohemian spa town, Teplitz.

Only one woman we know of satisfies these conditions. Her name is Antonie Brentano. But there is a problem. Antonie was married with children. In fact, she was in Prague, and subsequently Karlsbad, with her husband and youngest daughter. If Antonie was indeed the Immortal Beloved, it means Beethoven, the most moral of men, had an affair with her under the nose of her husband and while she was supposedly caring for her six-year-old daughter.

Bonnie and I talked about Beethoven and Antonie for hours, time after time. I needed the female perspective. I wanted to know how a woman like Antonie could possibly be attracted to Beethoven, who even his friends acknowledged was uncomfortable in female company, did not take much notice of how he dressed, and was even careless about issues like personal hygiene.

Bonnie taught me something of the subtleties of female behaviour. I will not claim that her insights in any way made me an expert, but I at least learned not to judge women's behaviour by men's criteria, to see things, as it were, through different eyes, if not exactly female ones.

But the single most illuminating moment came when, after a long conversation that began somewhere around nine in the evening and was still going strong in the early hours, I presented Bonnie with what I considered to be the clincher, the final proof that Antonie could not be the Immortal Beloved.

'Look,' I said emphatically, 'no woman who is away from home with her husband and daughter would have an affair. For a start, it would be too risky, and anyway, she wouldn't possibly be able to get away to have the affair.'

Bonnie said nothing; she simply looked at me and raised one eyebrow.

＊　＊　＊　＊

Bonnie has developed an obsession with tissues. Tissues and toilet paper. All neatly folded. Pockets stuffed with them. Handbag full of them. Piles of them around the flat. Bedside table stacked with neatly folded pieces of toilet paper. Why? I leak, she says. There's no evidence of it. Just all that paper, and fragments of it on the floor. I don't know how it gets there. It's too obtrusive to try and watch.

Every now and then, I freak out over it. You don't understand, she says quietly. But I do. There is nothing to understand. It is an obsession, caused by the dementia. Living with it is a nightmare. Not for her, for me.

Yesterday, when we went shopping, I was cruel to her, and it breaks my heart. The love of my life, and she now moves slowly and thinks ponderously, and somehow I seem to be blaming her for it. How can it be her fault? And yet I resent her for what's happening to her.

My biggest fear was that I would get this thing too, but Ian spelled out a bigger one. 'If you don't come to terms with it, you'll go before her. You're her primary carer,' he said, 'and she needs you more than anybody. She relies on you. If you go, she'll lose the person she needs most.' Great. From lover to primary carer.

I'm really aware of it now. A tightening across the chest whenever I find myself trying to cope with everything, organising this, organising that. One day – soon – that'll be happening and I'll just keel over. Then I'll be a fat lot of use to her, won't I?

I must come to terms with what is happening. Her world is shrinking, a neurological nurse explained to me a little while ago. Within that world, she is happy. So don't ask her to operate outside that world. Don't introduce new things. Stay inside her world with her.

Simple enough. Shouldn't be too difficult.

* * * *

Sometimes, looking back at those research trips, I marvel at the way things dropped into place for us. Time was never on my side. My holiday entitlement from ITN was spent at Tardan, writing. The research trips had to be fitted in over short periods. Mostly this was at Easter or other Bank Holiday weekends. It meant each trip had to be carefully planned, with a set of objectives to be fulfilled. At least, that is how it should have been. Maybe, if I had been a professional author with no day job, I could have planned it like that. In the event, each trip was haphazard, places visited chosen randomly. It should have been a catalogue of errors, Bonnie should have complained profusely. But she was at my side every step of the way, my good luck charm.

She was stoic as we walked the streets of Vienna hunting for Beethoven's favourite taverns (there are a large number, as you might expect for someone who almost certainly died of cirrhosis of the liver). We ate in countless seedy bars with Beethoven associations and she barely murmured a word of protest as I took in the atmosphere and imagined the Great Deaf One feasting at the next table 200 years before us. She was probably panicking when I mentioned that he lived at more than 70 addresses during his 35 years in Austria, but I didn't try to visit all of them. Honest.

I did drag her to the village of Gneixendorf, where his brother Johann had lived, and where he retreated in crisis in 1826. Through pure good luck, we stumbled across the very house, the very rooms even, in which he'd stayed, and Bonnie was mortified as I, journalistic instincts to the fore, marched in waving my camera and interrupted the current incumbents in the middle of their Easter Saturday lunch. Bonnie rolled her eyes to the heavens, but was right behind me as the owner showed us upstairs to the actual apartment Beethoven had stayed in. On the walls of the small living room were murals of the Rhine, which Johann had had painted to remind him of the river on the banks of which he and his brothers had grown up. It was at these murals that Beethoven gazed as he composed the last complete piece of music he was ever to compose. In all the research trips Bonnie and I undertook, all the places we visited, no single moment brought me closer to Beethoven than standing in that room, gazing at those same murals.

Bonnie relished my enthusiasm, but that enthusiasm masked a certain insecurity, which I articulated to her. Thousands of books have been written about this great artist, there are books of several hundred pages devoted to a single composition. What on earth could I contribute? What made me think I had something to offer that had not been said before? Always she met these doubts head on. 'You are not a musician, not a musicologist. Nor are many millions of people all over the world who adore Beethoven's music. You are writing for them, not the specialists.'

Ah my Bonnie, without your encouragement I would never have got past Page 10. You allowed me to fulfill my dream.

* * * *

I thought I had registered a small triumph. Bon has begun to put all the kitchen lights on when she gets up in the night, and leave them on. So they are burning for the best part of the night. I thought carefully about how to handle this. I waited until we were about to switch the bedroom lights out and go to sleep.

By the way, I said, nothing important, but when you get up in the night, try not to put the kitchen lights on. She looked bewildered. Did I? Yes, but don't worry, just try to remember. OK?

Next morning, lights on and burning hot. Next night, I tried the same approach again. She got a little short, denied she had put them on, but said OK. She got up at around 3am. I decided to check. When she came back to bed, I got up. Lights on.

Last night, brainwave. She went to bed first. I closed the kitchen door, then came to bed. I thought that if she saw it closed – we never normally close it – it would jog her mind.

Next morning, door still closed, lights off. Result.

At breakfast she said, 'By the way, did you lock the kitchen door last night?' I said, 'Er no, I definitely didn't lock it, I just closed it.' 'Why?' she asked, 'I wanted to go in to get something.' To turn the lights on more like, I thought. 'Yes, sorry,' I said, 'I don't know why I closed it. I won't do it again.'

What's the problem with living with kitchen lights burning for the best part of the night? So that's what we'll do. Sorry, planet.

We went to Bonn to see Beethoven's birthplace and then the house where he spent his formative years (now a hotel subtly named Hotel Beethoven). I showed her all the Beethoven sites, even taking the tram with her upriver to the Drachenfels, the mighty rock on the opposite bank of the Rhine which the boy Beethoven used to climb, and which he stared at through the telescope in the attic of the house on the Rheingasse.

Poor Bonnie. Over every meal she had Anorak John, yakking on and on about the childhood of Beethoven, when all she was trying to do was digest her food and enjoy her cappuccino.

Yesterday we had Sunday lunch with some very old friends, who live about an hour out of London. John and Jill. We've known them for 30 years or more. Went fine, with the usual caveats. Jill said at one point, 'I don't know how you are able to cope.' Made me feel a bit of a martyr.

That evening, Bon said that was a wonderful meal Peter and Marnie (our English friends down in France) gave us. I smiled, and because it was such an obvious mistake, had a go at correcting it. Not Peter and Marnie, I said. Can you remember who it was? She smiled, shook her head. I said we were with them just a couple of hours ago. Still nothing. I said gently John and Jill. She again looked confused. Glass of wine time, I said.

The good news is she didn't get angry, nor did I get frustrated. But I still haven't quite come to terms with not trying to correct anything. I must learn. Just go along with it, it's kinder.

One major source of regret on my part. Last time we saw Peter and Marnie in France, they told us they had found this wonderful apartment in Venice. They've stayed there once, and are doing so again. It's perfect, Marnie said, right on the Grand Canal. All we have to buy is coffee and breakfast, then lunch and dinner we eat out. We're going there again to charge our batteries for Christmas. Also John and Jill are off to Cape Town for Christmas and New Year.

Bon and I can't do that sort of thing any more. Sad.

There is a famous incident in Beethoven's life that encapsulates his stubborn and haughty character perfectly. In 1812, he was in the Bohemian spa town of Teplitz (Bad Teplice in the Czech Republic today). While there, he met the distinguished German poet Goethe, of whom he was a great admirer. One morning, as the two men strolled together through a park in Teplitz, the Empress and her retinue emerged from a bathhouse. Goethe took up a position on the path ahead of the Empress, and as she approached he removed his top hat, swept it low across his body and executed a deep bow.

Beethoven, by contrast, pushed his top hat firmly onto the back of his head, clasped his hands behind his back and strode defiantly away from the royal party. It was a calculated insult. Beethoven, man of the people, was having none of it.

Afterwards Goethe wrote to his wife that Beethoven was an utterly untamed personality. Beethoven wrote to his brother that Goethe fawned too much before the court. As far as we know, the two men didn't meet again.

Oh, to have witnessed it! There is a famous painting depicting the incident, and I had a copy of it alongside me as I wrote up the episode in the third volume of my trilogy on Beethoven's life. I wrote it, and rewrote it, and rewrote it again. Somehow it just never seemed quite right. Something was missing. Free as I was allowing my imagination to roam (within the constraints of the facts), I needed to see with my own eyes where this had happened. But how to do it?

Bonnie and I both worked from Monday to Friday and I'd used up all my holiday from ITN. It was late June, and I was already nearly a month overdue in delivering the manuscript to my publisher for publication in November.

Could we do it in a single weekend? Logistically it was just possible, but it would be a nightmare rush, and it depended on everything going exactly according to plan, no late flights, no car hire issues, no map-reading problems. What would Bonnie say? Would she agree to give it a try? What normal wife would give up a relaxing weekend at home after a hard-working week to go tearing around Bohemia in unrealistic pursuit of a fantasy? (Interestingly – and this is only occurring to me now as I write – it didn't for a moment cross my mind to go alone.)

I poured her a nice glass of wine, then explained the plan in as non-manic a way as possible, trying to make it sound the sort of thing you'd do any weekend.

'But that's crazy,' she said. 'What if ...? And if ...? I mean, there's no guarantee ...' 'You're right,' I said, 'it's a bit nuts.' Her eyes lit up. 'I'm game,' she said. 'Darling, I've told you before, you mustn't say that. It's not ladylike.' And I hugged her half to death.

* * * *

She remembers odd things, but skewed. Last summer – four months ago – I read a book about the fall of the French monarchy during the Revolution. One of the reasons that Marie Antoinette became so unpopular with the French was that, despite being married to Louis for several years, she was simply not producing an heir.

Marie Antoinette's mother, the formidable Empress Maria Theresa of Austria, decided to send her son, Emperor Joseph, to Paris to find out what was going wrong. It would appear that he persuaded his sister and her husband to allow him to watch them having sexual intercourse, because he wrote his mother an extraordinary letter in which he said words to the effect that Louis inserts his member in the appropriate place, lies on top of his wife for six or seven minutes without moving, then withdraws said member. Damn fool needs a good whipping, he adds.

Fascinating stuff, no? I read it out loud to Bon at the time, and we both had a good laugh.

Fast forward to yesterday. I did a massive Beethoven gig at the Wigmore Hall, launching a new edition of the piano sonatas. I was worried sick – had been for weeks – but I did my homework and it went OK.

Took Bon out to dinner, and said didn't they love that story I told about the pupil Beethoven was in love with, but she went off and married someone else who turned out to be impotent? 'Yes,' she said, 'and do you know what, he used to put it in and leave it there without moving! Can you believe that? Without moving!'

I've learned. I shook my head and laughed.

* * * *

Saturday morning. The flight to Prague left on time. So far, so good. We hired a car, and unlike every other tourist in the car park, drove away from Prague northwest into deepest Bohemia. By coincidence we arrived in Teplitz on the same day of the year as Beethoven – 5th July – 185 years later. Unlike him, it took us a comfortable two hours. We skirted round the thickly wooded Waldtor forest, where his carriage broke down. Again like Beethoven, we were unable to get a room in the main hotel in the town square. They directed us down the hill, at the bottom of which there was a small newly built hotel. In we went, just the faint stirrings of panic at the thought this one would be full too, but fortunately it wasn't.

I asked for a map of the town and, in our room, I unfolded it on the table and my heart sank. There were at least half-a-dozen splashes of green in the town of Teplitz, and a dozen more outside. Parks every-where. 'Why can't it have one bloody park?' I shouted in frustration. 'We only have tomorrow morning, there is no chance of going to them all.'

The next morning, it was Bon who came up with the solution. 'Beethoven was staying in a hotel down here, roughly where we are now, is that right? And Goethe presumably at the main hotel in the square, which we couldn't get into, yes?' I nodded. 'Well, Beethoven will have gone to see Goethe then, not the other way round.' I nodded again. 'So the likelihood is they'll have walked out of that hotel, into the main square. That's where the castle is, isn't it? So they'll probably have strolled through the castle into the grounds, then into the park. Is there a park behind the castle?'

I looked at the map. There most certainly was. The *Schlosspark*, the Castle Park. 'My God, that's it. You're right! That's where it must have happened.' 'That's the most likely,' she said, 'so we might as well start there.' 'It's more than just likely,' I said forcefully, 'it *has* to be right. It's obvious when you think about it.' She should have said, 'If it's so bloody obvious, why didn't *you* think of it, genius?' But she just gave a little smile.

The castle was more a palace than a castle, now a museum but formerly the home of a high-ranking nobleman, and it lined one side of the main square. We walked behind it, into the grounds, then out into the park. It was a large park, paths criss-crossing everywhere. In the centre was a pretty lake with fountains spraying up jets of water, which sparkled in the sunlight. I stood in the centre of the path we were walking along.

'Right, I am making a decision. I am going to base the incident here, right here. Look, there's a building over there. I will make that the bathhouse out of which the Empress and her retinue came. In fact, it looks as if that is what it was. Beethoven and Goethe were over there –' I gestured vaguely '– and let's say they hurried across the grass to this spot, and –'

If Bonnie and I had somehow been taking part in a Hollywood movie, at this point there would have been several shots of me, in close-up, blurred, turning this way, turning that, eyes opening wider and wider, and coming to rest on a small stone monument set into the path a couple of metres from where I stood. 'What's that stone monu –?'

I walked up to it and read the German inscription. 'At a spot close to here Beethoven, walking with Goethe, encountered the Empress of Austria.' I stepped back onto the path, and there in the centre of it was a plaque. 'On this spot Beethoven insulted the Empress of Austria.'

After the triumph of the *Schlosspark*, we drove to Karlsbad (Karlovy Vary today). It was where Antonie and her husband and daughter were staying, and Beethoven left Teplitz to join them there. Could the love affair have continued right under Franz Brentano's nose?

The little river, the arcade where Beethoven and Antonie must have walked and talked of what might have been, the small houses along the riverbank, retain their original charm. You just have to ignore the hideous oblong tower block that stands above the municipal baths – a gift to a grateful people from their Communist rulers. Today the town is a magnet to German day-trippers from across the border, as well as film aficionados who come to the annual film festival.

We lunched beside the river, took a leisurely drive back to Prague airport, and were back in our flat by mid-evening. The next day,

Monday, in the newsroom, my programme editor asked me if I had had a good weekend. 'Yeah, fine,' I said. 'Lovely, wasn't it?' he said, 'did you manage to get out much?' 'Yeah,' I replied.

* * * *

When she went to bed last night, she put three glasses of water on a small tray. I said gently, 'Shall I take one of those off? You don't need three.' She looked a little bewildered, but said OK.

I came to bed 10 minutes after her, and there were four glasses of water by her bed.

This morning we got up and I said, Shall I take those glasses of water (still full) to the kitchen, or do you want to keep them by the bed? She said yes, take them, someone asked for lots of water, I don't know who, that's why they're here.

I need my Mum and Dad more than I ever did. I want Mum to wrap her arms round me and tell me everything will be alright, and I want Dad, who was a surgeon, to give me advice.

We need our parents when we're kids. When we're adults, we think we can do without them. Then we really need them when it's too late.

Chapter 9

Bon came home from work one winter's day in early 1997, flushed with excitement. 'Chuck is giving me – us – a present to celebrate my 10th anniversary as his PA.' 'That's great,' I said. 'What is it? A diamond ring?' 'Don't be silly. He's sending us on holiday for a fortnight.' 'Really?' I was a bit surprised, even maybe a little shocked, as if he was entering a bit too intimately into our lives. 'Where are we going? Do we get to choose, or is he making the decision for us?'

I could see a slightly mischievous look in her eye. 'He is making the decision for us. But I don't think you'll object.' I knew Chuck owned a hotel outside Limerick. Beautiful though Ireland is, much though I love it, it would not at that moment have been my first choice of holiday resort. Somewhere a little more certain to get the sun would have been better.

'Pour me a glass of wine,' she said. I obliged. She clinked my glass. 'What would you say to Phuket and Bali?' Ever seen a man open his mouth when it is half-full of wine? She leaned forward and kissed me. 'You've taken me to so many places. Now it's my turn to take you.'

Chuck had a major share in a hotel in the Thai resort of Phuket, as well as a golf club with individual thatch-roofed cottages on the Indonesian island of Bali. We were going to spend the best part of a week in each, and to cap it we would spend a few nights at the Mandarin Hotel in Hong Kong, where we would be looked after by a Chinese artist Chuck knew.

Well, I mean. Talk about the trip of a lifetime! It began with an upgrade from British Airways (my contribution) on the flight to Bangkok, and a bottle of champagne from the steward as a parting gift. A limo awaited us at Bangkok airport, allowing us to crawl through the manic morning rush hour in air-conditioned luxury. We had one night in Bangkok before flying down to Phuket, where the general manager of the most beautiful beach-side hotel I had ever seen personally greeted us and showed us to a luxury suite. We enjoyed sea, sun and sand. We swam in the hotel lagoon, which snaked through the grounds, lined with tropical plants and Thai statues. We ate grilled fish lifted from the water just hours before. We drank cock-tails. We took a Thai massage together, lying on adjacent mattresses as two tiny women worked our muscles, cracked our joints, and walked on our backs. We helped each other back to our suite, hobbling slightly and swear-ing we would never have another Thai massage.

On Day Three, the general manager put his driver and car at our disposal, with instructions to end the day at a restaurant on the other side of the island. That evening we sat on an outside deck, thick tropical foliage forming a roof. It was dusk. A thousand candles provided the only light, the sea underneath us stretching into the distance, cruise ships twinkling on the water. I think they were the most romantic surround-ings we had ever eaten in.

Bonnie wore a light-coloured chiffon top. She looked like Grace Kelly. If it had been a movie, I would have brought a diamond ring out of my pocket, got down on one knee and proposed, to the sound of a thousand violins. We looked at each in disbelief. Once, it seemed a hundred years ago, the very thought of ever being together at all had seemed beyond reach. Here we were, not many years later, in Thailand, man and wife. We talked little, both marvelling at what had happened to our lives.

✳ ✳ ✳ ✳

I was about to leave for work and couldn't find my keys. They should have been in the top lock of the door. They were nowhere. I searched every pocket, my briefcase, my coat. Finally I gave up and said, Love, could I borrow yours, you're not going out today? Sure, she said. She reached into her handbag and found hers immediately. I had a brainwave. I don't suppose there's another set in there, is there? She rummaged a bit, and out came my keys. 'I don't know how they got there,' she said. 'We'll never know,' I said smiling.

Then she said something very strange. She looked at me in a questioning way. 'When you go now, you know, as you're about to, as you do every day, do you, do you go to the same place each day and do the same thing, or do you do something different every day?'

John struck dumb and silent. What do I say? How do I answer that? I have been going to the same place and doing the same things for the last two years, namely presenting the news. Before that, I did the same thing at another place for more than 20 years.

She still looked questioning and confused. I knew I had to stay calm and answer her rationally. Well, you know, I said, I go to the same place and do the same things each day. She looked more confused, so it wasn't going well. But obviously the news changes each day, so the bulletins change. Relief on her face. That's what I mean, she said. It changes. Absolutely, that's the nature of news. She smiled. She was happy. I think somehow she realised she had got herself into a bit of a pickle, but between us we found a way out of it.

And just in case you think it's always as bad as that, when I got home, I poured us out some wine. I took a gulp – that first taste bursting in my head and slipping down my throat as if my life depended on it. God, I said, don't let anybody ever tell me I mustn't drink any more wine.

'No,' she said, 'what is it they say? Wine – the elixir of life.' My jaw dropped. Before I could stop myself, I said 'That's brilliant!' Patronising, true, but I really was stunned. She gave me a cheeky look. 'Well, I'm not stupid, you know, I went to Cornell University.'

* * * *

The next day we flew to Bali and as we emerged with our baggage we saw a small dusky man holding up a huge sign which read 'Bonnie Suchet'. 'Now that's what I call impressive,' I said to her. 'We arrive at a small airport on the other side of the world, and there is your man waiting for us.'

He drove us to the country club, where the manager personally escorted us to our private cottage, set in its own grounds, with an outdoor swimming pool and indoor whirlpool. He showed us into the bedroom, a circular room with a straw roof rising conically to a point high above the bed. There was a sheet of thin gauze suspended below the roof. I asked what it was for. He smiled. 'Geckos. There are geckos in the roof. They like the straw. You don't want gecko do-do to fall on your face while you sleep.' Correct. We laughed about 'gecko do-do' for months afterwards.

Bali is an extraordinarily spiritual place. The men have coloured markings on their cheekbones to ward off evil spirits. Saucers with lighted candles are placed everywhere – there was one on the corner of our swimming pool – for the same reason. Food is blessed before it is cooked. We drove high into the tropical forest on the slopes of the island's volcano. Everywhere there is a pervasive sense of calm and spirituality. For four days we were alone together in our cottage. Just the two of us. You can imagine.

From the blissful peace of Bali to the bustle and roar of Hong Kong. The Mandarin, with its rich colonial history, the Star ferry across to Kowloon, up to a small dodgy room to bargain for fake Rolex watches for the boys. I called into the ITN bureau, saw the preparations being made for the handover of the colony to China in a few months' time. It would be the rainy season. Hadn't they thought of that? It wouldn't be at all surprising, our producer moaned, if the whole ceremony took place in a tropical downpour. (I smiled months later to see the Governor, Chris Patten, stand head bowed as the Union flag was lowered, drenched to the skin, large droplets of rain dripping off the end of his nose.)

We met up with the Chinese artist who was Chuck's friend. 'Have you ever had a Chinese meal?' he asked. 'Er, well yes, a few times,' I said, wanting to add 'thousand' after 'few'. 'No, a *real* Chinese meal,' he said. He took us to a restaurant where they clearly knew him, and we sat at a specially prepared table. He didn't order, the food simply came.

A large bowl was brought, full of water, with shrimps swimming lazily in it. He saw my puzzled look and raised a finger to forestall any question. A second bowl was brought, larger, covered with a high lid, a hole at its centre from which rose clouds of steam. He pulled up his sleeve, expertly lifted a shrimp from the warm water and dropped it through the hole in the lid. He waited a moment, smiling to both of us, lifted the lid, spooned the shrimp out, shelled and ate it.

We sat wide-eyed. He repeated the process, handing us each a peeled shrimp. I had never tasted a fresher, more succulent, shrimp in my life. Bonnie and I quickly overcame any squeamishness and allowed him to feed us. The rest of the meal passed in a gastronomic blur. It truly was a meal to remember.

… I looked up just now from the laptop. Bon had come into the *séjour* on her walking tour of the house. 'Do you remember when Chuck sent us on a trip to the Far East?' I shouldn't have asked, but I wanted to know. She frowned. 'The Far East? I don't understand.' I smiled and let it go.

… I am writing this the following morning. By total coincidence, there was a cookery programme on television last night set in Bali. The memories it brought back! The grey statues of gods alongside the road, the dense foliage and small shops lining the road on the lower slopes of the volcano, the offerings in saucers, the sheer beauty of the smiling women. We sat watching it together. At the end, in a matter-of-fact voice, I said, 'Bali is beautiful, isn't it? Have you ever been to Bali?' She looked slightly bewildered. 'No,' she said.

* * * *

It's Christmas night, and it has been a dreadful day. I have finally got Bon to bed and come to the computer to pour it all out. In a nutshell, I completely lost it. But completely. Worst breakdown for months. As always, it was a build-up of minor issues. Decided I couldn't tackle turkey, so cooked an M&S ready-to-put-in-the-oven piece of beef. I slightly overcooked it, but she said she didn't mind. I asked her how many slices, she said two, and didn't eat a single mouthful of it. No problem.

I realised in the afternoon she needed to wash out her stockings for tomorrow, when we're going down to my son Damian's in-laws. She's got dozens of pairs, but these are the only ones she wears. I told her to take them off, put her slippers on, and we'd wash them. She said fine. I went back to the sitting room and she came in with the stockings on and wearing boots.

Later I raised the stockings issue again. She again said fine, but when I asked her to take them off, she became thoroughly confused. It took a while, but she finally did it. I realised it would have to be me who washed them, which I did.

Washing-up time. Would you wash up? Yes, of course. It'll need detergent, I said, pointing to the detergent, because we've had red meat. I know that, she said. She rinsed everything and dried it all up. No detergent.

I lost it. Xmas night. Great. Well done, John. Finally she said, 'I'm going up to bed.' We live in a flat. Why do I let these little things get to me? She went along the corridor via the toilet, and within a couple of minutes came back via the toilet. Small pause, then to the bedroom again via the toilet. The carpet outside the bathroom is strewn with tissue fragments like so much confetti. Same in the bedroom. Why? How?

Tonight I've taped over the button of the bathroom heater. It would have been on for eight hours last night if I hadn't got up and turned it off. The kitchen lights? They'll be on all night. Sod it.

I really am on the brink tonight. We're with family tomorrow. I only have to make sure she dresses appropriately. If the stockings have shrunk, we're fucked. And I've got to wrap Xmas presents. And sort out bottles of wine and champagne to take. And book the car.

Easy.

I hate Xmas. I really hate Xmas. I am already dreading next Xmas. I suppose it can't be much worse than this one. Oh yes, it can. It doesn't bear thinking about. Peace and goodwill. Yeah, right.

* * * *

Bonnie retired from her job of a lifetime in 2001, and Chuck gave her an amazing send-off in his Limerick hotel. People she had known for years only on the telephone flew in from around the world. How embarrassed she was to be the centre of attention. At the retirement dinner, she made that speech and looked stunning. She wore a two-piece, red silk suit we had chosen together. The silk was shot through (I think that's the expression), and buttoned down the front with large black velvet buttons.

She was laden with gifts, perhaps the most precious being a small book the office had put together, in which colleagues recorded their memories of her. I have that book in the study at home. In the years following her retirement, I would regularly take it from the shelf, leaf through it, read her passages, and watch her blush. I can't bear to look at it now.

But I must, to show you I am not her only admirer. It is a tall, thin, hard-covered book, with Bonnie's name inscribed in gold on the front cover. Here are some quotes from it:

'Your svelte presence has been a benign influence on all of us. It will be hard to get used to your absence, but your spirit will remain with us …'

'You are a real American lady, softly spoken, beautifully dressed, courteous, and gracious …'

'You are beautiful, intelligent, discreet, and unflappable, an island of sanity in a sea of chaos ...'

'Bonnie, you walk with quiet elegance ...'

'Without exception you have drawn personal praise, gratitude, respect and admiration for what you have done, how you communicated, how you managed. You have always been graceful, pleasant, positive, supportive and encouraging – even when getting the blighters to bugger off ...'

'Some people come into our lives and quietly go. Others stay for a while, leave footprints on our hearts and we are never the same. And thus it is with you, dear Bonnie.'

They all, of course, wish her a long and happy retirement.

If she knew I was revealing this, she'd kill me. Right, I need to go into a corner with a box of tissues.

I had my own little retirement celebration planned for her. I booked us first class on Eurostar to Lille, where I had reserved a luxury suite on the top floor of one of the city's best hotels for a long weekend. The bathroom had a double-sized jacuzzi. We made the most of it, we most certainly did. We did leave the hotel once or twice. Well, you've got to eat, haven't you?

A few days after we returned to London, Bon was unwell, very unwell. I had to call a doctor. It was one of those infections women get that are usually knocked on the head by a course of antibiotics. Only it was worse than usual. In the event, it was the beginning of a round of visits to specialists, a series of difficult investigations, and antibiotics for the following two or more years.

She has never fully recovered. What caused it? We don't know and will never know. For a long time, I blamed the jacuzzi, what we did in it, and the fact that water that remains in pipes can become infected. Maybe, maybe not, probably not, in fact almost certainly not. What then? Who knows. All I know is that from that day, Bon suffered from pain and discomfort down below, which has never fully cleared up.

✳ ✳ ✳ ✳

At dinner last night, I said, 'Super-douper'. Monika laughed, then blushed. 'What means this word douper?' she asked, a glint in her eye. I said I had no idea, it doesn't really have a meaning, it just rhymes with super. She said, 'In Polish it means bottom, arse, and is very rude.'

Bon, quick as a flash, without a syllable wrong, said 'Supercallifragilisticexpialidocious.' Shock!

✳ ✳ ✳ ✳

Could the day have begun worse? Shower, darling, then I'll shower. I go to the computer to do my morning checks, e-mails, bank statements, news websites. Fifteen minutes, 20, no sign of Bon. I go into the bedroom, she's fully dressed. You haven't showered? No, I'm just about to. But you're dressed. I know, I'll get undressed and go into the shower. There's no time now. We have to leave for the clinic. You stay dressed and I'll shower.

I shower. As I come out, she is in her dressing gown waiting to go in. No, darling, you need to get dressed. I know. Come on then, we'll go to the bedroom together and get ready. Yes, fine. In the bedroom, she takes her dressing gown off and underneath she is fully dressed.

I leave the bedroom and have a truly bad moment. I nearly bang my head against the wall very hard indeed. I stop myself, but I can't stop the tears of frustration.

We go to the neuroquack for a cognitive test, and it's pretty dreadful. Year, month, day, date … nothing. Name as many animals as you can. Dog, cat, giraffe … that's it. How many words can you say that begin with f? Furry … that's it. Take 7 away from 92. Er …

A year ago she scored 22 out of 30. Today it was 16 out of 30. I call that pretty dramatic, but the quack said actually it's within the parameters of what you would expect. Yeah, well, I still call it pretty dramatic.

At the beginning of the session, the quack asked Bon how things were, and so on, and she just said fine, fine, fine. He then took me away for a private chat, and I opened up. He agreed that the best of it all was how totally benign she is, how she accepts everything I suggest or say. I told him about Monika, what an enormous help she was, and how I had given up work, retiring from newscasting for the second time a few months before at the end of 2007. He said I appeared to have things well under control, had a structure in place, should stop beating myself up when I have bad moments, and I was obviously doing a very good job.

Doesn't feel like that sometimes.

Bon's brothers and their wives visited us at Tardan in 2001 and Bob loved it so much he decided he wanted his ashes scattered in the local market. Their visit was also significant for a breathtakingly daring decision we took.

The large L-shaped barn attached to our farmhouse had slowly been falling down over the years, and the old attic over the house, which used to store straw, had become home to dozens of unwelcome small creatures. The year after buying Tardan, we had the downstairs renovated, so we could at least move in. Now something more was needed. How many times had we discussed this, standing in the dusty old barn and imagining a beautifully restored farmhouse? Countless times over the years. But now we had to make a decision. If we did nothing, one solid fall of snow (rare, admittedly) would bring the barn down.

We found a builder (not easy – the French love new homes but are not so keen on doing up ruins, which they leave to the Brits). We discussed it all at great length with Bon's brothers and wives. The attic would become a vast master bedroom. It had a low roof and no windows. The builder said he would raise the roof and put in two huge dormer windows. 'Your bed will go here,' he said, pointing to the dusty back wall, 'and one of the windows will be there, opposite. Because you are English, you will drink tea in bed, and you will be able to see the valley through the window.' I told him that was impossible, but he smiled knowingly. The small downstairs bedroom would become a study, where I could write about the Great Dead Deaf One. The barn for the most part would be pulled down, and a large covered terrace created. Where the barn joined the house, the right angle of the L, the builder would create two more bedrooms and a bathroom upstairs.

It was like a dream, what we had always envisaged. There was the teeny problem of money. It would be very expensive. But when have I ever let that stop me doing anything? Another trip to the bank, that was all. The more wine we drank, the more it seemed a really good plan. We could then truly spend our retirement here, in the beautiful house we had always imagined.

Bon's family left, wishing us luck with the project. I kept insisting my mind was not yet fully made up. The following day, I came up with an elaborate charade. I summoned a board meeting. Bon and I sat at the oak dining table. I opened a bottle of wine and declared the meeting open. I read the agenda: *To make a decision on whether to proceed with the renovation, Stage Two*. I threw it open for discussion. Bon listed all the reasons why we should go ahead. I countered with reasons why we should not. We discussed and drank, drank and discussed.

Finally there was no more to be said. But there was a technical issue to resolve. We needed to vote. Since there were just two of us, it was possible there would be a tie. 'In the event of a tie,' I said authoritatively, 'We will then, er, there will be, er, we will have to open another bottle of wine.' Bon nodded seriously. The moment had come.

'In honour of the French love of formality,' I said, 'and remembering that they lost the Battle of Waterloo, we will take the vote in reverse order. All those in favour of not proceeding with the renovation, that is to say the renovation should not be proceeded with, please raise your hand …' Bon set her jaw, and kept her hands firmly on the table. I raised my hand to my face and stroked my chin, but no further. 'No votes,' I said. 'All those in favour of proceeding with the renovation, that is to say the renovation should be proceeded with, in accordance with the terms heretofore discussed, and contained within the papers put to this meeting, please raise your hand.' Bon smiled and raised her hand. I did the same.

'I declare Project Tourterelle [named for the lovebirds that nest each year in our eves – I know, I know] is to go ahead.'

In January 2002, the builders demolished the old barn. By the summer, we had the house of our dreams with the large upstairs bedroom in the old attic. And yes, for years afterwards I would bring Bon a cup of tea in bed in the morning, and we would gaze out over the valley.

But Bon's health was not good, and I was worried. She just could not shake off the gynaecological problems. One summer's evening, I was standing at the gate talking to the builder. Bon came out of the house and walked towards us. I had never seen her so pale and drawn. I put my arms round her immediately, to try and inject some warmth and strength into her.

I am sitting at the same oak dining table now, writing this, and Bonnie is walking uncomprehendingly up and down the kitchen. It is a truly beautiful summer's day. She should be out on the terrace – she would have been in days gone by, expertly tanning her front and back for just so many minutes – but without me she will not. I will stop now, and go outside, safe in the knowledge she will come out with me.

Chapter 10

I am a Romantic, capital R, unreconstructed. You hadn't noticed? Really? Well, I am. I can't tell you how many surprise moments I have given Bonnie over the years. Birthday or Christmas presents, a sudden meal out, a concert or West End show. You name it, I have planned it, and delivered it as a surprise. I have always succeeded, because Bonnie is not a suspicious person, not someone who is constantly trying to divine what is going on, or what lies behind this or that piece of behaviour, or this or that remark.

But now, in early 2003, I was planning the surprise of surprises, the *ne plus ultra* of surprises, the ultimate, the surprise that would redefine surprises. Why early 2003? 27th April 2003 would be the 20th anniversary of the date on which, 20 years before, Bonnie stood at Baltimore Washington International in her straw hat with the paper flowers round it (I can see it now, hanging on a hook here in Tardan). She sat nervous as a fawn on the drive into the city, I opened the door of the bedsit in Washington, she walked in and did that twirl. The first day of our life together.

I intended to mark it, and in an unforgettable way. But how? I could book one of the best restaurants in London run by one of the new masterchefs. That would have been problem solved for your average romantic. But I am *not* your average romantic.

Next I considered Paris. Eurostar there on Friday. Book the best hotel – no, the most intimate one – on Saturday walk the city, show her where I worked as a young Reuter correspondent covering the 1968 revolution, intimate candlelit dinner, Sunday more of the same, then a special dinner on Sunday night, the anniversary day itself, Monday Eurostar to London.

But then I thought, 'Paris? Yawn.' All right, it wasn't bad, better than an average romantic would come up with, but I am an *über*-romantic, the King of Romantics, the Holy Romantic Emperor. And so I pondered on. The crucial element was the Sunday night dinner. I had already decided I wanted a photograph of that dinner, a photo to go into our album, alongside the original one from 1983.

So, where could we have that dinner?

It came to me in a moment of inspiration. Venice, of course. The most romantic city in the world, a city we had never been to together. In fact, we had often discussed the fact that if we had not bought our French farmhouse, we would have made many more trips to Italy. So, Venice. Decision made.

The Big Gig. I got my Lifetime Achievement Award in February 2008 and Bon and Monika came along. It went very well. Bon, bless her, was confused about what the event was, what we were doing, when I was going up for the gong, and so on, but as always was thoroughly benign and amenable. She wanted to go to the loo at all the wrong times, but Monika was on hand to take her.

Journalists from my past had been invited without me knowing, so the evening was emotional and thoroughly wonderful. They all knew Bon from years back, and greeted her warmly. She looked absolutely stunning, and loads of people commented on it. I have brought back an engraved piece of glass, which has made me a very happy man indeed.

In the event, it was to be my Bonnie's last public outing.

I contacted a travel agent that specialised in short city breaks and asked for their brochure. I wanted us to be away from the bustle of the city and considered the Lido, but he had another suggestion. The north of the main island, an area known as Canareggio, would be really quiet in April. There was a beautiful hotel there, which he recommended highly. It used to be the residence of the French ambassador and had a lovely garden, something that was rare in Venice. Many of the rooms looked out on the lagoon, and the hotel had a motorboat that would take us to the Rialto Bridge in the city centre free of charge, whenever we wanted.

Well, what would you do? I said yes, please book me a double room, with lagoon view if possible. I added that the trip was to celebrate a special anniversary, and when the agent got back to me he said we had been upgraded to a junior suite in a separate small building at the bottom of the garden, right on the edge of the lagoon. Attaboy, I said.

So now to book the flights. I was idly flicking through the Venice brochure when it fell open at a particular page and the words *Venice Orient Express* leapt out at me.

I didn't think twice. I booked us on the Venice Orient Express leaving Victoria Station on Thursday 24th April, arriving Friday afternoon, in the Hotel Dei Dogi in Canareggio for five nights, returning to London British Airways club class on Wednesday the following week.

The problem now would be keeping it secret. But this was not dinner in London, or even Paris. It was complicated. Women like surprises, I knew that, but not too much of a surprise. I remembered years before an ITN cameraman telling me how he had booked a surprise trip for him and his wife in January. She was thrilled, packed her cotton dresses, several bikinis and suntan lotion. He took her to the Shetland Islands.

* * * *

This morning I got up to make us tea as usual. Stay in bed, I said, I'll bring tea up to you. I came up five minutes later to find she was dressed, with her beret and scarf on. I wasn't totally surprised (except for the beret and scarf), said nothing, just got into bed myself. She looked slightly confused, then without saying anything took off her scarf, skirt, boots and stockings and got into bed.

There we were in bed, drinking tea. I was just in boxer shorts, Bon was in a cashmere sweater and beret. I guess if someone had taken a picture of us, it would have looked oddly funny. It even brought a very brief smile to my face.

I read the small print on the Orient Express tickets rather late in the day. Passengers were not permitted to bring large suitcases on board. Large suitcases should be handed to the steward on boarding the train at Victoria station. Passengers should bring a small bag containing enough for a single night, which they were permitted to take to their compartment.

That settled it. I couldn't keep it a secret. I knew women liked surprises, as I said, but this threatened to be a surprise too far. Wouldn't Bonnie be happier knowing? It would give her something to look forward to, as well as avoiding any packing mishaps. Separate a woman from the clothes she would like to wear, and you are asking for trouble.

So I planned an elaborate charade. First, I told her we were going to Venice. She yelped with delight. Then, in true John style, I carried it from the sublime to the ridiculous. 'Unfortunately all the direct flights are booked. So we are stopping over at another hotel on the way.' 'All right,' she said, 'that's not too bad.' 'Yes, but you know how you don't like heights, winding mountain roads, all that kind of thing?' She looked slightly apprehensive. 'The hotel I have booked us into is in the Alps, at the top of a mountain. We're going to be lowered down to it from a helicopter. And as the helicopter only has a small hold, we have to pack an overnight case to take with us. We'll be sending our main cases on ahead.'

I don't know what came over me. Neither did she. She got the joke immediately and laughed. I realised then the folly of what I had done. I had mixed fiction with reality. I hurriedly said, 'No, I mean it, we really do have to pack overnight bags, because the, er, helicopter –'

I repeated this mantra over the next few days, until she believed me about the overnight bags. Why did I keep up the helicopter and Alpine hotel fiction, when it was clearly nonsense and she knew it? I don't know.

One night shortly before we left, she made a classic Bonnie remark. I said to her, 'Tell me, darling. Here I am planning something truly complicated for our anniversary, and you haven't even asked me what it is. Why?' 'Because it's your surprise, and I don't want to spoil it for you.'

Now, be honest, how many wives would say a thing like that? Some months later, after it was all over, I was telling a good friend about the elaborate charade, and she said to me that if her husband had tried to pull a stunt like that, getting her to pack in different cases without telling her why, she would have put her hands round his throat and slowly throttled him until he told her. As any wife would. Not my Bonnie.

And so for reasons I cannot explain (other than that my romanticism is incurable), the Orient Express journey remained a secret. The day before our departure, I went down to Victoria station and scouted it out. I didn't want to be fumbling round looking for directions on the day itself. There was a side entrance to the station that led on to Platform One and there, 20 or so paces down the platform, on the right, was the check-in office for the Orient Express.

We packed for the trip together. I found myself making the decisions for her about what to take. It seemed natural, since I was keeping so much secret. But I was aware it was something I was starting to do naturally, and she acquiesced in happily. Now, of course, I look back on that rather differently. It was as if she knowingly abrogated the responsibility of packing to me, as she has done ever since.

* * * *

We watched a programme on telly about memory, and how it develops. The final section was about Alzheimer's. It featured a man who was diagnosed in his early fifties. A gentle, grey-haired chap, whose hobby is jogging. He knew the route well and his wife was not concerned about him getting lost, but he didn't know which kitchen cupboards held the plates, and who the grandchildren in the family pictures were. He smiled about his condition, and said he wouldn't let it get him down. He had a firm, strong-willed wife. The spouse becomes like that. Inevitable, when you're the one making all the decisions.

But what was really interesting was that Bon sat watching the whole programme, didn't react at all to the section about the A-thing. At the end, she just said that was really interesting, and we all went to bed.

* * * *

The day dawned: 24th April 2003. I continued the ruse after the taxi driver dropped us at the side entrance to the station, telling Bon that we had to wheel our cases across and catch the Gatwick Express. We turned right onto Platform One. I let her go just a half step in front of me. We drew level with the Orient Express office. 'Darling, stop a moment, would you? I need to adjust this strap –' She stopped. I slipped the overnight bag off my shoulder. I stood the two cases upright. I stepped towards her. She saw the almost evangelical look on my face. I took her by the shoulders, kissed her on the lips, said, 'I love you, my darling Bonnie,' and turned her to the right. 'Look up,' I said. She looked up, and saw the large sign that proclaimed VENICE SIMPLON ORIENT EXPRESS. I propelled her gently forward.

She turned to me and gasped. 'We? … Are we? … Is that? …' I nodded, eased her forward, picked up the bags, and led her into the check-in room. She had tears rolling down her cheeks and so did I.

The young woman behind the check-in desk saw these two adults, obviously a married couple, walking towards her in tears. I read the look on her face. 'Oh bugger. A domestic.'

We reached the desk. 'He didn't tell me,' Bonnie said between sobs. 'You mean –' the young woman replied, 'he didn't tell you?' 'No,' Bon said, 'it was a surprise.' 'A surprise!' the woman gasped, and tears came to her eyes. The three of us cried and laughed in unison.

It's my birthday today, March 29th. To be honest, I had forgotten. Monika remembered. When I came down for breakfast, she gave me a card. Bon looked a little sad at first, then smiled and wished me happy birthday. We had mentioned it a few times over the last few days, because it's Jean-Pierre's birthday today too and we're all going out to dinner together. I don't mind that Bon didn't know. It's really minor.

It was all so wonderful. Dinner on the train as we left Paris. Complimentary champagne 'because, sir, we understand it is a special anniversary.' Our bunks, of course, were one above the other, which led to an elaborate ritual of strangers meeting on a train and finding themselves sharing a compartment …

We awoke the next morning to a view that might have been a Hollywood backdrop. The majestic and jagged Alps, sweeping hill pastures populated by the most contented cows I had ever seen carrying large bells round their necks, small villages and onion-domed churches.

We sat drinking strong coffee and marvelling at how beautiful Central Europe was. I spoiled it slightly by warbling, 'The hills are alive'.

An image remains strongly in my mind. The train stopped somewhere outside a Swiss village. There was a path alongside the railway track, houses behind it. A small boy in smart grey school uniform, satchel on his back, was walking along the path to school. I don't know why it struck and stuck – maybe because it was a scene that must have taken place, with variations, for hundreds of years, and probably would do for many more.

By lunchtime we were passing through the mountains, to emerge into the greenness of northern Italy. As we travelled south the sun strengthened, and by late afternoon we were passing through the lower, flatter, damper plains north of the Golfo di Venezia. Finally across the Ponte della Libertà from the mainland, onto the island of Venice itself, and clanking to a halt in Santa Lucia railway station.

A private motorboat awaited us and whisked us around the north of the island, down a small canal to the front of our hotel. We were as excited as children. We walked in and our jaws dropped. It was the most beautiful hotel we had ever seen. Chandeliers sparkling with highly coloured glass made just across the water on the island of Murano, everywhere glass, cabinets, ornaments. Almost immediately, I spotted in one cabinet a glass statuette of two lovers in an embrace. Silently I decided not to leave Venice without one. What better commemoration of our visit could there be?

We walked to the reception desk. An Italian woman with a delightful accent welcomed us. I mentioned what the travel agent had said, that we were to be in a junior suite, and she said, 'No, no, you are in the Presidential suite, with our compliments.'

I gasped. She told us to leave our bags, came out from behind the desk, and we followed her out into the garden. Down a gravel path through highly scented bushes and flowers, towards the small building at the bottom of the garden, on the edge of the lagoon. We entered it and climbed the circular staircase to the first floor. She opened the door and ushered us, not into a room, or even a suite, but into an apartment. A large sitting room, elaborately furnished and dominated by another splendid chandelier. Above, a bedroom which projected out over the sitting room. Two bathrooms, one on each side of the sitting room. One was merely luxurious, the other contained the largest whirlpool bath I had ever seen.

For the next five days, we were young honeymooners again. We saw the sights, we ate freshly grilled fish, we photographed ourselves on the Rialto bridge, we toured churches, we saw great works of art. The highlight, of course, the most important element of the trip, the *raison d'être* of it in the first place, was the anniversary dinner on 27th April. It was a Sunday, so I played it safe. No searching for restaurants that may or may not be open. I reserved a table in the beautiful restaurant of our beautiful hotel. I told Bonnie that we would have a glass of *prosecco* in our apartment before going down for dinner at eight o'clock.

She started getting ready early evening (late afternoon, actually). At one point, she was standing in front of a mirror in a cream satin gown, putting on some eye make-up. She was a stunning sight. I whipped out my camera, but she turned and said, 'Do you want me to be on time, or not?' I clicked the shutter and captured a wonderful smile, a mixture of pure joy and gentle exasperation.

Both ready, we sat in luxurious armchairs, I opened the *prosecco* and poured. We clinked glasses, and I said, 'To us'. Then, as we had 20 years before, we toasted the future.

For a moment, I looked at her. The beautiful young woman I had fallen in love with had matured into a woman with a deep inner beauty that radiated from every pore. Her eyes sparkled and danced, her cheeks lifted by the upturned corners of her mouth into a permanent semi-smile.

I told her to stay there, and went to the chest of drawers against the wall. I opened the bottom drawer and pulled out a small box I had hidden under some clothes. I stood behind her and told her to close her eyes. I took out a necklace I had bought her and put it gently round her neck. She opened her eyes, held the pendant, and gasped. It was a small glass heart encrusted with diamonds, inside which a single diamond moved freely. I turned it in her hand to show her the reverse side was gold. 'Gold for daytime, diamonds for the evening,' I said proudly.

She looked up at me, her eyes moistening. I reached down and kissed her. At dinner I asked someone to take our photograph, and it sits in our album alongside its twin of 20 years before.

That necklace is round her neck now, as I sit here writing this. It is mid-morning and she is pacing the house. She has the diamond side showing, but she will get angry if I try to tell her about one side being gold, the other diamond, so I won't say anything.

In London. Took Bon across the road for dinner. Halfway through, she looked at me and said, 'Thank you for looking after me.' I said, 'I try my best, but occasionally I fail spectacularly.' She said, 'I haven't noticed.' It was a nice moment.

On our final day, we went to a glass factory on Murano. We watched a master craftsman demonstrate how to blow a smoldering globule of glass into a delicate prancing horse. In the shop at the end of the tour, there were endless statuettes of lovers, their faces fused in a permanent embrace, their bodies joined in a single length of sculpted glass. I told Bonnie I wanted to buy one as a memento of our anniversary trip. She said it was a lovely idea.

I looked along the shelves. The colours were strong. There was a perfect statuette made of pale green glass, which graduated from medium strong at the head to clear at the feet. Unfortunately it had the lovers reclining. I wanted a standing statuette. Their permanent kiss would be an everlasting reminder of our kiss that fateful night so many years before.

A young woman asked us in heavily accented English if she could help us. I nodded and said I was having trouble deciding. 'No, no, you must-a choose and we make-a for you.' My eyes opened wide.

We sat at a table with her and she got out an order book. We selected the size, the colour – graduated green – and then she said, 'We write-a on it-a for you. You choose-a ze words.' She brought down one of the statuettes from the shelf and showed me how the glassmaker could inscribe words on the top of the base.

What could be better? Barely able to contain my excitement, I told her I wanted 'John & Bonnie, 27th April 2003'. She wrote it on the order form, but spelled Bonnie's name wrong. I pointed it out. She scratched it out and corrected it. I wanted to ask her to start a new order form so there could be no confusion, but with her English and my Italian that was out of the question. It took her two or three attempts to write our London telephone number correctly, and even more to get our address right. I had a sinking feeling. I knew what I should do: choose a statuette from the shelf, take it to London and have it engraved there. But we had gone too far down the road to turn back. I gave her my credit card details, and told Bon that with any luck in a couple of weeks we would receive a statuette of the Pope or the Virgin Mary, with who knows what inscription on the base.

Our dream anniversary trip came to an end, we had our own personal motorboat trip to the airport, and we flew home club class. We walked into our flat, I closed the door behind us and took Bonnie into my arms. 'Would you have believed it, 20 years ago in our bedsit, that we would celebrate our 20th anniversary like that?' We stood, arms entwined, for several minutes.

✳ ✳ ✳ ✳

We had a family get-together yesterday, and it was amazing. Bon sailed benignly through it. She didn't know which were her grandchildren and which were mine, and she kept referring to her small grandson as she, but it didn't matter. I'm glad the whole family had a chance to register what was going on, and to meet Monika.

Around three weeks after we got home from Venice, I received rather a strange telephone call. It was a man's voice, he spoke in guttural, heavily accented English, and said he was calling from Hamburg in Germany. I was about to put the phone down, thinking it was a crank call, but he said, 'For you ve have a parcel, Ja? Ve vill send to you in London, Ja? I wish to confirm address.'

'Parcel? From Germany?' 'No,' he said, 've have parcel here, in Germany, but ze parcel it comes from Venedig, Venezia.' A lightbulb flickered in my head, then sparked to life. 'Venice, Venice? Yes, that's for us,' and I confirmed the address. He said we should receive it within three to four days.

If I had been worried before, you can imagine how I felt now. I told Bonnie to expect a parcel from Germany containing a statue of God knows what, intended for God knows whom, with an inscription saying God knows what.

The parcel duly arrived. Bon was out shopping, which I was quite pleased about. I would open it, uncover the disaster-in-waiting, get on the phone to the glass factory and try to sort the whole thing out before she got home.

I took a sharp knife to the packing tape, surlily removed the polystyrene bobbles and shredded paper protection, reached in and slowly extracted … the most beautiful piece of glass artwork I had ever seen in my life.

I cradled the statuette of the lovers in my hands. Their lips were joined forever, their bodies swept down in unison, the gentle green of the glass lending them a kind of eternal glow. On the base, perfectly inscribed, were the words *John & Bonnie, Murano 27.4.2003*, along with the name of the artist (there is no other word to describe him) *Caetano Tosi*.

I held the statuette away from me, stroked its shape, and placed it on the mantelpiece of our living room, where it stands to this day, an ever-lasting reminder of our anniversary trip.

That evening, we sat gazing at the statuette and reminiscing. I could-n't help talking about all the over-elaborate planning I had put in. 'Do you know?' I said, 'I nearly didn't tell you it was Venice we were going to.' 'Well, I'm glad you did,' she said, 'It gave me something to look forward to.' 'Yes, you're right,' I said. 'In fact, maybe I shouldn't have left it so late. Maybe I should have told you a couple of weeks earlier.' 'But you did,' she said, 'you told me before Christmas.'

I knew this was wrong, and it disturbed me, but only for a moment and not very deeply. Maybe I was the one who was wrong? But deep down I knew I wasn't. I put it out of my mind.

There is a problem, and it concerns Monika. We got up this morning and Monika already had coffee on the go. Up in our bedroom, I said to Bon this was exactly what I wanted to happen, that Monika would be up before us and get coffee going. Mmm, that smell. 'Bloody Monika, always Monika,' she said. I was stunned, but didn't say anything.

Breakfast was difficult. Bon said virtually nothing. Afterwards she cleared away. She always does that, as if to make up for not cooking. But what she does is rinse our mugs, then wipe them with a tea towel, making it pretty stained, then she puts the mugs into the dishwasher. This morning, Monika tried to stop her drying a mug, saying it was going in the dishwasher anyway, and Bon got very cross.

Monika said she liked coming down and opening the shutters, feeling the cool air. Bon couldn't understand what she meant. What shutters? Where? I don't understand. And she walked away.

Monika left the kitchen and I said to Bon, 'Why are you being so difficult today?' 'I don't want to talk about it.' 'Well, I have to live with it.' 'Alright, I'll tell you. It's bloody Monika. You seem to like her more than me. Always praising her. I feel left out.'

So all my efforts to make Bon realise just how much of a help Monika is being are in danger of back-firing. I told Monika what she had said and we both agreed I would stop telling her how pleased I was about everything she was doing.

Monika painted Bon's nails this afternoon, and Bon didn't stop praising her for ages.

In the autumn of 2003, we travelled to the US, back to Bonnie's old university, Cornell. She was on the university's Council, an honorary position which didn't actually involve any work, and there was a big bash to celebrate the appointment of a new university President.

By now the discomfort below was pretty much a constant thing. She had been checked out, again and again, but the medics could find nothing. She was on antibiotics, off them, on again. I was concerned about the trip, discussed my concerns with her, but we both decided it would be a shame not to go. In the end, I'm so glad we did, because it led to an unforgettable moment.

The highlight was a formal dinner, for which the gymnasium had been converted into a huge dining area, with dozens of round tables. At the pre-dinner drinks, amazingly and without it being planned, Bonnie met one of the women she had made that trip to Europe with over 40 years before. But that is not the marvellous moment I am referring to.

We moved into the hall, looking for the table to which we had been allocated. We found it, looked around, and I spotted a man of about our age standing four or five tables away. He was bald, kept looking in our direction, and seemed agitated. His wife (I presumed) was gesturing to him and pointing to us, as if she was encouraging him to approach us. Suddenly the man nodded, set his jaw, and walked towards us.

I nudged Bonnie, she saw the man, and gasped. 'My God, I remember him,' she said, an embarrassed smile coming to her face. 'He was, er, well, I think he quite liked me.' That made me smile, and the man clearly picked up on the fact that we were both smiling, and he smiled too. He reached us, said hello to Bonnie, and shook my hand.

There was a kind of stilted conversation, then his wife joined us. She knew Bonnie too. It transpired they had both been students at Cornell at the same time as Bonnie. The man had fallen in love with Bonnie, had pursued her unsuccessfully, and had then started dating the woman he had gone on to marry, who was now recounting this story, much to his embarrassment. 'So you see,' she said, 'he couldn't get Bonnie, so he had to settle for me.'

She spoke totally without rancour, and all four of us were laughing. The man pulled me slightly to one side, as the two women carried on talking and reminiscing. 'You are one lucky man,' he said unashamedly. 'I tried my best but it wasn't good enough. What's your secret?' I laughed out loud and said if I knew, I'd bottle it and offer it for sale. I remember saying to him that it was the biggest shock of my life when Bonnie told me she had fallen in love with me, and I was still trying to get over it. I had certainly given up trying to understand it. We both agreed there was no telling with women.

We rejoined the women, and Bonnie and the man's wife were exchanging numbers and addresses. The couple were planning to come to London the following summer, and we all agreed it would be great to meet up.

In the event, we didn't hear from them again, and we lost touch. I can't even remember their names, and there is no point now in asking Bonnie.

She had no health problems on the trip, which was a relief. When her term on the Council expired a couple of years later and she was asked to serve another term, it was by then out of the question. We didn't yet have the diagnosis, but her health was clearly a major issue. So that was her last trip to her old university.

I messed up good and proper last night, oh yes. At dinner, great food, good wine, relaxed at the end, and I was telling one of my interminable stories. Monika was listening with (feigned) rapt delight. Bon got up to go to the toilet. Fine. I carried on. She came back. I was still in full flow. Seconds later, she got up again and went to the toilet. Fine. I carried on. She came back. Got up again. I said no, this is the third time in five minutes. NO!

She sat down angrily. I said right, let's all go into the *séjour* and watch some news. I went in. Bon went to the toilet. I went to check she was in there, and banged my head on the cupboard so hard I nearly did myself (and the cupboard) damage.

She came into the *séjour* to join me. We watched. She said nothing. Finally I said, 'Why don't you go up now? I'll come up in a few minutes and bring you your pills.' Up she went. I followed, gave her her pills, and came back down.

By the time I went up 20 minutes or so later, she was in bed, the bedclothes pulled up, half asleep. I got ready for bed, turned off the lights, and got into bed.

5.30am, up she got to go to the toilet. Fine. I became aware of the toilet flushed, but no Bon. I heard footsteps out on the landing, a small bang here and there as if she was knocking into something. I put on the light and called to her.

She appeared in the doorway with relief. Phew, she said, I thought I had lost you. No, you're fine, I said, come to bed. Only then did I see she was fully dressed. When could she possibly have done that?

It took me a moment to work out what must have happened. She couldn't have got into her clothes when she got up to use the toilet – the lights weren't on. She must have got into bed last night fully dressed, and slept in her clothes. Why? Because she was in such a state after my outburst.

So it was almost certainly me who caused this latest bout of confusion.

I worked this out lying in bed early this morning, after telling her to take her clothes off, get into her nightie, and try to get another couple of hours' sleep. It began to rain heavily as I lay there, pounding on the tiled roof just a few feet above our heads. It matched my mood.

Chapter 11

There were three people in our marriage. Er, I will rephrase that. There were two people and a *thing* in our marriage. I have described how, starting some time after the Lille trip, Bonnie began to complain of pain down below, and how for a long time she was prescribed antibiotics. One day – I forget exactly when, but probably early 2004, certainly long before the dementia diagnosis – she announced she would never again sit in a chair without first putting a cushion down.

Cushion. Even now, almost six years later, the word gives me a pain in the chest. One of the doctors had told her you could get something called a Valley cushion, specially designed to be gentle in the middle to allow people with *that* sort of pain – primarily, of course, women – to sit in comfort. I ordered one on the internet for her.

This blue thing, carried in a brown leather bag that had been a freebie with some cosmetics, became a permanent fixture. She went nowhere, *nowhere*, without it. That bag, and its precious content, became an extension of her arm. Concerts at the Royal Academy, restaurants, theatre, friends' homes, anywhere, *everywhere*, along came the bag and out came the cushion. I used to look around in embarrassment as it was carefully positioned. You may say I should not have reacted like that, but I did. I hated *hated hated* that cushion, for being such a visible sign of all that was now going so wrong. And also, naturally, for what it was doing to the one thing we had always taken for granted in our lives – the amazing, incredible, unquestioned physical intimacy.

During this period, we did a constant round of doctors. All kinds of doctors, in all shapes and sizes. Urologist, gynaecologist, bladder-iologist (I made that up, but you get the gist), pain specialist, another pain specialist ...

In early 2006, she underwent a bizarre treatment, which I witnessed. A pain specialist said he would administer an analgesic directly to the area where Bonnie complained of pain – low down, around the bladder and urethra. I watched it happen. Bon was sedated, though not totally, lay on her front, and was positioned under the arch of an MRI scanner, so that it showed the whole pelvic floor area.

The specialist then got what looked like two extra-long knitting needles, with tubes coming out of one end, and inserted one in each cheek of Bon's bottom, positioning them with extreme care. He took me into the small room adjoining the theatre, separated just by glass. On a computer screen he showed me Bon's pelvic floor area, then pointed to the two knitting needles. I could see that the way he had angled them meant they were both pointing directly at the area where Bon complained of pain.

'Now,' he said, 'I will administer the analgesic, but before that –' he shot me a grin, went to a small machine in the corner, inserted a CD, and the opening chords of Beethoven's *Fifth* blared out. I took it as a good luck token.

I watched him back in the theatre open valves in the tubes, and saw liquid flow slowly through them. He hurried back into the computer room and pointed to two small veinlike white flows, which the MRI scanner showed. It was the analgesic fluid.

'See!' he said triumphantly. 'It is going to exactly the spot where she says she has the pain.' It was true. The thin white lines meandered across the screen towards each other, converging at exactly the right spot. 'That is a strong analgesic,' he said. 'There will be no more pain for possibly as long as several weeks, maybe months.' 'And then?' I asked. 'Then we will be in a better position to decide what to do next.'

It worked for 24 hours or so. Then out came that fucking cushion again.

Since then, I have taken Bonnie on round after round of doctors. Test after test after test, and they have never found anything, no cause for the pain, no explanation for her discomfort. I know now what I didn't know then: that it is, of course, the dementia. Her nerves down below are relaying a message of pain to her brain. The pain is real to her, but there is no cause for it. Ergo, there is nothing that can be done.

As for that cushion, in 2007, maybe 2008, we were leaving for the flight down to France. It was absurdly early, around 3.30am. We were both a bit groggy. I saw the dreaded brown bag underneath her dressing table. We walked to the front door and she forgot to take it. I decided to say nothing.

This was particularly cruel of me. As I said, the pain was real to her. That cushion had gone on every surface she had sat on for several years. Without it, she would be in agony. Still I said nothing, reasoning that if she had not forgotten it once before, then maybe something had changed, possibly for the better, to allow her to forget about it now.

Do you know what? She hasn't mentioned that cushion since. Not once. It went out of her life – our lives – as suddenly as it had entered. She still has the pain to this day, but it is a fraction of what it used to be like, and she no longer complains about it.

That pain, and the blue cushion, and the brown bag, were part of our lives for several years. I came to loathe them all, detest them all. Even now, I take shorter breaths just thinking about them.

Bonnie doesn't know this, but when we got back from France I quietly and triumphantly threw bag and cushion into the rubbish bin.

❋   ❋   ❋   ❋

A colleague of my Admiral Nurse Ian has put me in touch with a man roughly my age, who is going through the same thing with his wife. Both are retired headteachers and live in Bolton. Jan has been diagnosed with dementia.

By e-mail I told Jim about Bon's obsession with toilets and tissue paper. His wife is exactly the same. Extraordinary! Made me feel a lot better, and I hope him too. I have a feeling Jim and I are going to pour our hearts out to each other. Makes such a nice change from all the people who say they know just how I feel because they have a relative with Alzheimer's, then it turns out (always) they are in their eighties or nineties.

This new obsession of getting up in the night, getting fully dressed, and coming back to bed, is a perfect example of what I was told by a neurological nurse right at the beginning of all this. Bon has her world within which she is comfortable, and you have to enter it with her. So I no longer try to correct things, I no longer ask her why she has got dressed, I just let her do what she's comfortable with.

Maybe soon I'll get so used to it that I'll be able to sleep through when she does it, then I'll no longer fall asleep in the armchair in the afternoon trying to plough through the two-volume history of Poland I'm reading. Anyway, the obsession might suddenly go, or mutate.

The problem is when a new obsession comes along, and at first I don't realise it and get cross, before settling down and accepting it as part of her world. The new one is covering the bathmat with shreds of tissue paper confetti, then shaking it out into the bath some time during the night. It's really pretty trivial. Today is Day Two of doing this, and I got a little irritable when I saw it, but not nearly as bad as yesterday. Now I'll know to accept it, and keep my eyes open for something new soon.

It's a help for me to know that what I am having to deal with is nothing compared to my new friend Jim. At least Bon can still get dressed on her own, even if it is in the middle of the night. His wife Jan certainly cannot. Again that knowledge is tempered by the realisation of what lies ahead.

The cushion and its bag remain consigned to history. Bon has also stopped carrying a handbag. That is good too, since it was crammed full of nothing but tissues. And while I think of it, the three million glasses of water by the bed are also history. Obsessions mutate.

If you had told me six months ago that the cushion would go, I simply would not have believed it. So getting dressed in the middle of the night is a pretty small price to pay.

Had a chat with a woman called Joy, who works for a charity called *for dementia*. We met at her office in Camden at 3pm and went across the road for a cup of tea. After telling her about life with Bon for what I thought was half-an-hour or so, she said she ought to get back. It was a quarter to five!

She reinforced what Ian has said. Do not feel guilty, and get out more. Also, stop denying this is happening, and feel good about telling people when you need to. She asked, 'What do you think Bon would want, if you could ask her?' I said she would want me to do whatever was best for me. 'There you are,' Joy said. So obvious really, but you need someone to point it out. She said I am grieving at having lost Bon. It is true. I have lost her. I can't think of that without the tears coming.

The fantasy author Terry Pratchett has gone public about being diagnosed with a rare form of Alzheimer's. Margaret Thatcher's daughter has revealed her mother has dementia. Charlton Heston has died of it, as did President Reagan. There really is no telling, is there?

Sir Terry has donated half a million pounds to Alzheimer's research. Deep down inside me, there is a cynic gene. It's pretty dormant most of the time, but it has been getting a bit of a workout recently. While I applaud your generosity, Terry (if I may), I wonder what it will achieve? I have been making notes over the last year or so, and if you believe what you read in the papers, not only could you have saved your money, but Alzheimer's would be history by now.

There follows a small sample of 'Suchet's Miscellany of Alzheimer's Remedies, As Gleaned From The Daily Press [with comments by the compiler]':

… A blood test the makers claim can detect Alzheimer's and Parkinson's up to six years before they take hold is being developed, and researchers at Aberdeen University claim omega-3 oils, found in nuts, seeds and oily fish, can fight Alzheimer's. The blood test is in its early stages, and larger tests need to be conducted before it can be confirmed as being helpful. As for the omega-3 oils, for people without the crucial ApoE e4 gene [yes, that's the well-known ApoE e4 gene], the oil made no difference.

… A simple eye scan could soon be used to detect Alzheimer's. It's all to do with [yes, those well-known] proteins called amyloid plaques. An American-based company is due to carry out clinical trials later this year.

… New research shows that tomatoes [yes, humble old tomatoes] could be used as a vaccine against Alzheimer's. Scientists have genetically modified tomatoes to create an edible vaccine that fires up the immune system to tackle the disease. It works by attacking the toxic beta-amyloid protein …

… Doing brain exercises can actually increase your chances of developing Alzheimer's. Those little brain-testing machines that sold so well last Christmas can become so addictive that users neglect to do physical exercise, and scientists believe regular exercise can help prevent Alzheimer's disease by stopping the brain shrinking …

… A British GP has developed a high-tech helmet that sent one man's dementia into reverse by bathing his brain in infra-red light twice a day. Dr Dougal stresses that a full, clinically controlled trial will be needed before his anti-dementia helmet can be licensed for public use [yeah, right] …

… Being married halves your risk of developing Alzheimer's, say researchers. A study shows those who develop close companionship in midlife have a 50 per cent lower rate of dementia than those who don't. In fact, those who stay alone after divorce have a threefold risk of developing Alzheimer's in later life. [My grateful thanks to the Karolinska Institute in Stockholm for that.]

[Wait, there's more.] The Alzheimer's Society says anyone can take steps to cut their risk of developing Alzheimer's. 'The best advice is to eat a Mediterranean diet, exercise regularly, and don't smoke.' [In other words, behave exactly as Bon has done all her adult life.]

… A drug that holds back the ageing process, prevents cancer, heart disease and Alzheimer's, could be on sale within five years. The drug is made up of chemicals that mimic resveratrol, a compound which is found in the skins of red grapes …

It really doesn't stop, does it? And my cynic gene tells me it's all bollocks. Oh, to be proved wrong. The truth is simpler. Whether or not you are going to get Alzheimer's, or any other disease of the brain, or for that matter the heart, kidney, liver, breast, lung, prostate, colon, bowel, or any other part of the anatomy, is quite simply a lottery.

On 28th January 2009, I sat in the elegant palm-treed atrium of the Landmark Hotel in Marylebone in central London, about 100 yards from our flat. I was with two women, Barbara Stephens, chief executive of the charity *for dementia* which develops and supports Admiral Nurses, and Rhonda Smith, the charity's communications consultant.

We were discussing whether the time was right for me to 'go public' about Bonnie's dementia. This was an issue that had been on my mind for some time, something I'd been struggling with for a couple of years at least. It was almost three years to the day since we had been given Bon's diagnosis.

My Admiral Nurse, Ian, had said to me several times that if ever I felt ready to speak about Bon's condition in public, to do so would raise the profile of dementia and be a help to other people in my position, other carers. I told him I wasn't ready. How could I be? First, I had to come to terms with the fact that I had gone, in an agonisingly short time, from being Bon's lover to being her carer, from being the sole and adored lover of a woman of such compelling beauty and grace that she was, to me, a goddess, an angel, to being in effect a nurse and home help.

There was another aspect that worried me deeply. If I went public, would it be a betrayal of confidence? It seemed to me that Bonnie didn't know that she had dementia. Yes, she had been sitting opposite the neurologist when he delivered the diagnosis, but she didn't react. We had watched programmes about the disease on television and she had never remarked on it. Furthermore, she had never asked me if there was anything wrong with her, or could she have some sort of illness that the doctors had failed to diagnose? Given that she never fretted or seemed concerned there might be something sinister going on, I certainly had no intention of undermining this by telling her otherwise. If, to put it bluntly, she was happy in her ignorance, then let her continue that way. Given that, did I have the right to reveal it on her behalf, without her knowledge? My instinct said no.

Ian said that's fine, you must feel under no pressure, you must wait until you are ready.

The purpose of the meeting with Barbara and Rhonda was to brief me about an event the charity was holding at the Ritz Hotel in three weeks' time, on 17th February. It was being thrown and organised by the Lord Mayor of Westminster, Louise Hyams, on behalf of *for dementia*, the charity she had chosen to support officially during her one-year ceremonial term of office. Around 200 people would be invited, whom the Lord Mayor and the charity believed might offer both money and influence to improve the help and support on offer to carers around the UK, particularly the training and provision of Admiral Nurses.

Would I like to attend, they asked? There would be photographers and possibly reporters there, and if I was uncomfortable with that I should feel under absolutely no pressure. If I felt it was something I would like to be involved in, I could choose my level of involvement. I could be a guest, pure and simple. I could mingle with other guests or not, and if my inclination was not, the charity would make sure I was protected. If, on the other hand, I decided to use the event to go public, they would love me to say a few words.

The Lord Mayor, whose mother has dementia, would host the evening. The novelist Joanna Trollope, as a long-standing supporter and patron of the charity, would make the keynote speech. What was lacking, they explained to me, was someone to say what it was like actually caring for a partner with dementia.

'There is a perception that this is a disease of the elderly. It is, but it is more than that. There are a lot of people out there in a similar position to you, caring for a partner in their fifties or sixties, and there is nobody for them to turn to,' said Barbara. 'If ever you were to decide to speak out about Bonnie, there would never be a better time.'

'All right,' I said, 'I'll think about it.' Pause. 'I've thought about it. I'll do it.'

'John, if you do decide to speak in public about Bonnie, I think it will be big,' said Rhonda. 'There will be a lot of interest. A lot.'

I felt instinctively she was wrong. I was a journalist, with more than 40 years' experience. I knew what was a story and what was not. This, I felt sure, was not. But how to say it in a way that did not sound patronising, condescending, or aggressive even?

'I don't see it that way,' I said. Silence.

* * * *

A little under three weeks later, I was sitting in the *for dementia* office doing an interview with Jane Dreaper, BBC radio's health correspondent, about Bonnie's condition. It was the first time I had ever sat and talked to anybody like that, other than Ian. I was fine to begin with, but the moment I said the words 'my Bonnie' the tears came. It is simply a fact that I have always called her 'my Bonnie', both to her face and to other people. It has always seemed totally natural.

Jane was sensitive and kind, comforting me and being gentle. Of course, that made it easier to give in to the tears. There was no chance of a stiff upper lip. I did the interview and was told it would be broadcast on the *Today* programme on Radio Four the following week, on Tuesday, 17th February, the day of the *for dementia* reception at the Ritz.

The next Sunday, I sat in the self-same Landmark Hotel, talking to a feature writer from the *Daily Telegraph* about Bonnie. As with Jane, I felt that familiar sense of betrayal. I explained that to the journalist, Elizabeth Grice, hoping she would include it in the article she was going to write. I didn't want anyone to think I was comfortable about making Bonnie's condition known.

She was sympathetic, in a feminine sort of way, which was comforting, but also distressing. Unwittingly, by being so concerned for me, she breached the defensive wall I had built around myself, as had Jane. It wasn't long before I was wiping tears from my eyes. I was talking about my Bonnie to a stranger, and she intended to write an article about her for the newspaper. What on earth did I think I was doing?

I slightly comforted myself with my journalistic instinct that it wasn't really much of a story, and there was a likelihood the BBC wouldn't run the radio interview, and the *Telegraph* would drop the article. Rhonda had told me the intention was for both to run on the morning of the 17th. There was also the possibility of a live interview on BBC TV's breakfast programme, though that hadn't been confirmed.

Of course it hadn't, I wanted to say, because this wasn't a story. I e-mailed the family on Monday to warn them there *might* be a piece on Bon on BBC radio and in the *Telegraph*, but I doubted it. Rhonda called to confirm the BBC TV interview. That didn't change my conviction, based on a lifetime's career in news. This was not a story.

* * * *

Barbara said she would like to meet Bonnie, having heard so much about her. She came to the flat and we sat having tea together. Bonnie was easy and relaxed. Barbara chatted to us and we joked over whether I should do a parachute jump to raise funds. I helped Bon out a couple of times, identifying boys' wedding photos on the side tables. Other than that, she took part in the conversation and was on good form.

After an hour or so, I took Barbara into the dining room for a private chat and she immediately said how lovely Bonnie was, and what a wonderful relationship we have. Then she said, 'She's very impaired.' I gasped. I simply had not seen it. I had grown so used to intervening, helping out, covering up, that I simply had not seen it.

In fact, that is the complete opposite of what usually happens. When old friends who know of her illness meet Bonnie for the first time for a while, they always say how well she is, how amazing, how pleasantly surprised they are. That can be quite frustrating. You feel like saying, *If you only knew.* But Barbara is a professional. She saw what I didn't.

* * * *

Tuesday 17th February 2009. It is three years and two days since we got Bonnie's diagnosis. I had to get up early, shortly before six o'clock – the BBC was sending a car for me at 6.30. I went into the bathroom, ran the taps to shave, and switched the radio on as the pips went for six o'clock and the *Today* programme began.

The familiar voice of John Humphrys – the man who, when he was a BBC reporter and I an ITN one, had been my rival in Rhodesia shortly before independence – began with the headlines. The first one was something about the banking crisis and credit crunch. The second was: 'The journalist and broadcaster John Suchet has spoken movingly of his wife's struggle with dementia.'

My head sank down. I cried large tears into the basin. I could not control myself. My shoulders shook and I sobbed my heart out.

I showered and dressed, looked at Bon lying peacefully in bed, unaware that around half a million people were about to hear me talking about her. I kissed her on the forehead, hoping she wouldn't notice the shiny dampness in my eyes. 'I'm going out to do some interviews for the charity I'm working for. Stay in bed, get a little more sleep, I'll be back later.' Did she ask where I was going, what interviews, why? No, she just half-smiled and nodded.

I left the block and opened the door to the newsagents' on the street. The morning papers were piled on a table immediately inside the entrance. I gasped out loud. There was a large picture of Bon and me on the front page of the *Telegraph*. 'John Suchet's secret heartbreak,' it said. The *Daily Mail* had the same picture on its front page. I couldn't stop the tears. This was ridiculous. I had to get a grip.

I bought the papers and read the pieces in the car on the way to the BBC. They were sensitively written, very sympathetic, stating my reluctance to speak out and my doubts over whether I was doing the right thing. There was not a word of criticism, thank goodness. If there had been, I think I would have thrown myself out of the car.

I can't remember much of what I said to Jon Sopel on *BBC Breakfast*. The points I wanted to make were that Bon didn't know she had dementia, so I couldn't talk to her about it, as I could if it were cancer, that I didn't know how I would have managed without the advice of Ian and it was scandalous there were no more than 60 or so Admiral Nurses in the whole of England and Wales (none in Scotland or Northern Ireland), that Ian had explained to me that the welter of emotions I was experiencing were because I was in effect mourning my loved one, going through the grieving process for someone who was still there, and that I felt that in speaking out I was betraying a confidence about Bon and that made me feel guilty.

I remember at one point, as the tears welled, putting my hand to my face, thinking, 'Damn, this makes me look so stupid, they'll freeze it and say I broke down,' and at the end Jon Sopel reaching across and touching my arm. It was a lovely gesture of comfort, from one of my own as it were, but it made me cry. Fortunately the camera had cut away by then.

I went back into the hospitality room, where Barbara and Rhonda were waiting for me. They had tears in their eyes and both gave me great big comforting hugs. I just cried and cried. Had I ever cried so much in such a short time? I couldn't believe how utterly unable I was to control my emotions. This had never happened to me before, ever. I had cried my heart out when my mum died, my brothers and I had hugged each other, sobbing together. Then we started to talk about the good times, the good memories, and soon we were laughing through our tears at the remarkable woman who had been our mum. This was different – I was crying my heart out over a woman who was lying in bed at home, or maybe by now eating breakfast.

Thank God that's over, I finally said. I felt I needed to put it behind me. Bon was out there now, in the papers, on television and the radio. Now I wanted it to stop. In the next hour, my mobile rang time after time after time, as did Rhonda's. By the end of the day, I had done more interviews for the BBC, as well as ITN, *Channel 4 News*, Sky TV, local radio stations around the country, other newspapers, national and local.

I spoke about Bon time after time after time. It was getting easier in the sense that my thoughts were slightly more coherent, but was I better able to control my emotions? You would think so, wouldn't you? But I couldn't. This was my Bonnie I was talking about. Not some loved one who had died, but my Bonnie, waiting back in our flat for me.

The final event of the day, of course, was the one that had persuaded me to go public in the first place – the reception at the Ritz. It was a glitzy do, attended by the great and good, who had been invited both by the Lord Mayor and the charity. I was pretty much the centre of attention, since I had been all over the airwaves all day long and practically everyone there had seen me on one programme or another. That didn't make it any easier, and my eyes were permanently misty. Joanna Trollope spoke movingly; so did the Lord Mayor Louise Hyams, who announced she was going to do a skydive to raise funds for the charity. Then it was my turn.

Which do you think is easier: sitting in front of a television camera with an earpiece in your ear telling the news to around five million people, or standing up in front of two hundred or so and speaking about your wife's dementia? There is, of course, no contest.

There was a nice personal note. My penfriend, Jim from Bolton, was there. It was the first time we had met. In early e-mail exchanges, he had told me if ever we met I would recognise him easily because he was a dead ringer for Brad Pitt. Angelina Jolie, he wrote, would soon be given the opportunity to transfer her affections away from her high-maintenance husband and transfer them to him. I raised an easy laugh by pointing him out to the guests, and declaring that as well as the task of looking after his wife, he had the added problem of having to cope with his own delusions.

So I spoke about Bonnie for the umpteenth time that day, told the guests that she was at home with no idea I was speaking about her, pleaded the case for more Admiral Nurses, and ended up in tears. Again.

Afterwards I met a man and a woman of around my age, and was told that without them there would no such thing as an Admiral Nurse. They were Peter Levy and his sister Jane Jason. It was they who had the idea to train and develop mental health nurses and name them in honour of their dad – Admiral Joe – and who then founded the charity to act as the official body supporting them. Both have been awarded OBEs for their charitable work. Jane explained to me that the aim was to establish Admiral Nurses across the country. With a rather sad look, she said it had been something of a struggle – there were no more than 65 of them, and they were only available in a few pockets in England and Wales. Then she said, 'You have done more for this charity and Admiral Nurses in a single day than we have been able to do in 20 years.' I stared at her in disbelief. It was a humbling moment.

At the end of the evening, the Lord Mayor asked me where I lived. I told her Baker Street. 'I live in St John's Wood,' she said. 'Why don't you let me give you a lift home?' I accepted gratefully, and found myself gliding home in the back of the mayoral limousine, two chauffeurs in the front, and clutching a huge bouquet which had been presented to the Mayor and which she insisted I give to Bonnie. A surreal end to an extraordinary day.

It went on for several days more. I was interviewed on *GMTV*, the Alan Titchmarsh show, *Richard and Judy*, and others I can't remember. *This Morning* tried everything to get me, but we just couldn't fit it in. *The Sunday Times* wanted an interview, websites wanted interviews. And each time it looked as if things were beginning to calm down, in came more e-mails and letters. Between us, my agent and I received over a hundred letters and more than a thousand emails. I hadn't known before how many people across the globe log on daily to the BBC News website to see what is happening in the world. As they logged on, there was I, 'speaking movingly about his wife Bonnie's dementia' and I received e-mails from China, South Africa, the US and Canada.

Bonnie, bless her, had become a global phenomenon. I had well and truly put her 'out there'. Thank God, in all the letters and e-mails there was not a single word of criticism. Overwhelmingly, people were thanking me for speaking out, making the plight of carers known. At last someone is speaking up for us, they said. At last someone is talking about how difficult it is to care for a loved one, when you can't even talk about their dementia with them. Also, how do I get the services of an Admiral Nurse? Is there one in my area?

I did interviews with local radio stations in Scotland and Northern Ireland. Interviewers in both places were shocked to learn that there were no Admiral Nurses in their country. The one from Belfast was rendered almost speechless (not a very good idea for a radio interviewer). When he regained his composure he said, Right, we here at BBC Radio Belfast will start a campaign to train and provide Admiral Nurses in the province, and he asked me who they should get in touch with. I told them the charity that trains and provides them is *for dementia* and he said they could expect to be called. I thought, Yes, I know journalists' promises, having made one or two of them myself in my long career. They will forget about it in half an hour, move on to other stories, and that will be that. But they did not. As I write, they are in touch with the Department of Health, and waging a campaign to make Admiral Nurses available to carers of dementia sufferers in Northern Ireland. [Inevitable update. March 2010: there are still no Admiral Nurses in either Scotland or Northern Ireland.]

Did speaking out make it any easier for me? Most certainly not. In fact, the contrary. The final interview in the diary was with the *Tonight* programme on ITV. The actor Kevin Whately was making a programme about dementia, based on the problems he had encountered caring for his mother, who had the disease. He wanted to interview Ian and me together. I was pleased he wanted to speak to Ian – the more publicity for Admiral Nurses, the better.

The interview began well. I was making the important points I was by now becoming more used to making, and after a while Kevin turned to

Ian. Then it was back to me. I began again, the sentences flowing, and suddenly, quite suddenly, I opened my mouth and nothing came out. The word I had formed did not emerge. My mouth gaped, my eyes filled up with tears, and my head sank down. I whispered, 'Enough, I've had enough, I don't want to talk about it any more'. I felt Ian's hand on my arm and heard Kevin say, 'That's fine, that's fine, don't worry.'

In the car on the way home, Ian said, 'John, you don't know how much you've done this week to help carers.' I genuinely couldn't see it. Why? How? All I have done is talk about my Bonnie, tell people how this illness has changed her, and say a little about what it is like to handle the situation. Still, for me, the overriding sensation I felt was of guilt at having spoken in public about Bon, with her having no idea I had done it.

'This is the first time anybody has spoken out on behalf of carers, told what it is like to look after someone with dementia, how little help there is out there, and how much more there needs to be.'

Had I? Had I really? Had I done some good? Looking back at it now, it was obvious I had, but somehow I still had to get out from under this cloak of guilt and look at the positives that could come from what I had done.

Then Ian said something that I will remember for the rest of my life, that I repeat to myself like a mantra day after day, whenever the black dog settles on my shoulders. 'Thanks to you and Bonnie, dementia care in this country will never be the same again. You have changed it forever.'

In an instant, I saw that could be Bonnie's legacy, through me. If I could somehow tell the world what she was like, what this relentless disease has done to her, the effect it has had on her, me, our relationship, how it has turned me from lover to carer, how it has robbed her of her past, our past, how this disease, this vile unwanted thief, has robbed us both of our future, the future about which we used to talk so much, which we had so optimistically planned, joyously waiting for old age to envelope us so we could be alone together, right to the end … If I could do that, would it improve the lives of carers, and therefore of sufferers too?

If that were the case, it would mean that Bonnie herself would have helped countless numbers of people struggling to cope. Thousands maybe, even possibly tens of thousands. What a legacy that would be for a woman with the kindest heart and most loving soul it is possible to imagine!

Chapter 12

By now, Monika had become an integral part of our lives. She did the food shopping, cooked, cleaned, took care of the laundry – in fact, did everything Bonnie used to do so effortlessly. She also took much of the strain of caring off my shoulders. If Bon left something in an odd place, if glasses of water were stacked on a tray, tissue fragments scattered on the carpet, dirty plates back on the shelf, clean ones in the dishwasher, whatever, she quietly corrected it.

She also eased the emotional strain on me. Bonnie had developed a new obsession, or rather a variation on an old one. Frequent visits to the bathroom had become more than frequent, occurring every few minutes or so. One day, I decided to count them and gave up at around 30. Early on, I took to eavesdropping, because I needed to know if it was a real need or not. If it was, then it could signify something that might require a visit to the GP. I quickly established that was not necessary.

I don't know why I let it get to me. Maybe the fact that we lived in a flat, that I couldn't escape it, had something to do with it. In any case, it began to wear me down. I discussed it at length with my Admiral Nurse Ian. He said the obvious thing, that if it was doing her no harm, if she seemed to derive comfort from it, then I should simply let it glide over me. I knew that, but it was a help to hear it.

Monika said the same thing. More than that, she took over eavesdropping duties. We developed a basic sort of sign language. If Bon went and there was a result, Monika would give me a smiling thumbs up. It wasn't long, of course, before there was an added complication, and it is something every carer has to deal with at some stage. If there were times when Bon vanished into the bathroom with no result, there were also times – not many, admittedly, but even just once is stressful – when there was a result when she *didn't* vanish into the bathroom. Once again, Monika was on hand to put things right.

In May 2009, Monika was planning to go to Krakow for a fortnight to have some major dental work carried out. 'Why don't you and Bonnie come and join me for the second week?' she suggested. She said the clinic was providing her with an apartment which, given what was happening to Bon physically and mentally, would be a lot easier to handle than a hotel. Also, her family lived in a small town about three hours' drive from Krakow. We could go and meet them. I had serious reservations. Bonnie's health was clearly deteriorating. The travel alone would be stressful, never mind staying in a strange place. But I liked the idea of meeting Monika's family. It would be nice to tell them how easily she had integrated herself into our lives and how hardworking she was. There was the added attraction of a trip to the heart of Europe, to a country I loved and which Bonnie and I had already visited twice before.

It began badly and got worse. First, my elderly mobile phone decided to end its days in Krakow. Funny, I lived practically my whole career without the benefit of a mobile, yet to be without one for even an hour now feels as if I have lost a vital organ of my body. Just a touch more seriously, Bonnie was dreadfully confused. The apartment was alien to her. There was a corridor with rooms off it, not unlike our London flat but on a smaller scale. She soon took to pacing the corridor. The toilet was at the opposite end to the bedroom, beside the kitchen, and it became clear that she was unable to find it. I stepped in and helped. She was angry and confused. On the first night I got her to bed, the process of getting her into her nightie more difficult than I had known. She was clearly distressed. The next morning saw the inevitable consequence of the confusion over the location of the toilet.

We walked the streets of this ancient capital of Poland, its medieval beauty breathtaking to behold. We passed the café where, on our last visit a decade or so before, I had taken a lovely picture of Bon in sunglasses, taking a rare sip of beer. There was no point in drawing attention to it. She was confused and uncooperative, more so than I had ever seen her. Where are we? Why are we here? I'm tired, I don't want to walk any more.

At the end of the first day, we fell into a restaurant. My enthusiasm at being in Poland surrounded by so much history was boundless and I tried to convey some of it to Bon. She was unreceptive, picking at her food and obviously unhappy. I tried to chivvy her along, but she didn't respond. As we left the restaurant, Monika gave me a stern look, her jaw set. I wondered what it meant. Back in the apartment I found out. Bonnie's personal hygiene routine had collapsed. I needed to shower her (there was no bath) while Monika put her clothes into the washing machine (thank God, there was one of them). In the shower cubicle, she shouted and flailed. I had to leave the sliding doors open so I could help. The floor flooded. Finally I got her out and dry, almost having to fight her to get her into her nightclothes, and at last into bed.

The next evening, she again lost control, this time in the apartment. I was at my wit's end. I just wanted to energise us all, *Star Trek* style, back into our London flat. There was something else on my mind. The following week was a heavy one for me. I had agreed to take on two engagements, both charitable, which required me to make speeches. The second, for my own charity, was a major event, the launch of a programme for people with dementia called *Music for Life* in the presence of its royal patron. I was the keynote speaker and I was worried sick about it.

By mid-week in Krakow, I was beginning to feel unwell, but took no notice. We were due to visit Monika's family on the Friday. By then, I was feeling very unwell. I felt sick and had a worsening headache. Monika rang her family and told them we would come on the Saturday instead. By Friday afternoon, the sickness took hold to such an extent that when

Monika suggested calling a doctor, I did not demur. The doctor checked this and that, told me I had a touch of gastroenteritis, and prescribed a cocktail of tablets, seven different kinds in all. I took them that night and again in the morning. I began to feel a lot better. I told Monika we would leave after lunch for the drive to her family home. The original plan had been to go by train, but time was now tight so we took the more expensive but much quicker option of a taxi. Just as well.

I downed the tablet cocktail again at lunch, and at around three o'clock we left Krakow in a people carrier with three rows of seats, bound for Monika's small home town of Radomsko, via Katowice and Czestochowa. As soon as we set off, I began to get sharp pains in my lower stomach. They came in waves, every 30 seconds or so. Instead of slowly getting better, they rapidly became worse. After 20 minutes or so, the pain was a searing wave that almost made me cry out. Monika saw my distress, told the driver to stop and asked me if I wanted to stretch out on the back seat. I said yes. We set off again, but within minutes the pains became agonising. I feared my appendix had burst and poison was seeping across my lower stomach. Each time the wave of pain reached its apex, I expected to lose consciousness. It was unbearable. By now I was crying out, my face contorted. Yes, yes, man pain, but this was not, this was real.

We pulled into a roadside café. I fell out of the vehicle and clung to the side of a table. With each wave of pain, I threw my head back and cried out loud. Monika spoke rapidly to the café owner, who replied urgently, gesturing with an outstretched arm. There is a hospital nearby, she said, and I think we should go there. I knew she was right. My concern was that I might well be summoned by the Top Man before we reached the hospital. I had not once in my entire life known pain like it.

We pulled up outside the hospital and the driver procured a wheelchair. Into the emergency room and I was manhandled onto an operating table. There was some shouting in Polish as Monika explained what had happened to me. She told me the doctor said I must remove my signet ring, the one with Bonnie's and my initials on it. A nurse wiped my arm and I winced as she jabbed a needle into my vein and connected it to a drip. A young doctor in green overalls opened my shirt and yanked my trousers down. He started tapping my abdomen, moving gradually lower, all the time asking 'Hurt? Hurt?' No, I said, until he reached my lower stomach. He tapped and I screamed out loud.

Through my pain, I saw him smile. I thought maybe I was hallucinating, but he really did smile. If this were a movie, the next thing I would see would be a scalpel glinting under the operating table light. In fact, he diagnosed a spasm in my colon and was able to ease it – thankfully – with some dextrous manipulation rather than surgery.

'Had the pain been caused by the cocktail of pills?' I asked. He said no, and warned that the problem was likely to recur.

I went to see a specialist on my return to London just to check things over and he agreed with the diagnosis of colonic spasm. 'Did you feel under pressure at the time?' he asked, 'under strain?' My head sank down. Pressure? What's that? I just looked at him and nodded. 'You must take care of yourself, you know. Your body gives you warning signs.'

Point taken, but there is one other lesson from the Polish hospital incident, and it weighs more heavily on my mind than anything else. Bonnie was there with me the whole time, in the emergency room, just a few feet away as I lay screaming with pain, as the nurse attached me to a drip, as the doctor went about his business. Her face was blank, uncomprehending. She never once touched me, or offered a comforting word. At one point, when I was recovering fast, but still on the bed and attached to the drip, she looked at me with surprise. Oh there you are, John, I have found you. There was never even a fleeting look of distress on her face, this woman who once told me she would give her life for me if she had to (and I assured her of the same). It is comforting, of course, to know that I caused her no anxiety. At the same time, it reduces me to tears to realise just how much she has lost.

* * * *

My head feels as if it is about to burst. Really, as if my brain is pushing against my skull and the whole lot is about to explode. It's the build-up that always does this to me, usually of trivial things that just mount up, and a final one that threatens to bring everything crashing down. It has been a very difficult couple of weeks. Bonnie is getting worse. Her confusion is now acute. She turns the wrong way in the corridor of our flat. She doesn't know which meal of the day we are eating. She still hates getting dressed and undressed, or being made to have a bath.

There is something else. Personal hygiene, difficult before Krakow, dreadful in Krakow, now appears to have broken down completely. This is distressing for the person suffering it and it is distressing for the carer. It is distressing if it is happening to your grandparent or parent, so try to begin to imagine how distressing it is if it is happening to the person you live with, your partner, your lover.

Let me tell you a little something about Bonnie and her personal care routine in the past. On Sunday afternoons, she would do what she called her weekly 'service', which involved washing her hair, filing and varnishing her fingernails, and trimming her toenails. If it were summer, she would insert a weird white spongy contraption between her toes, which would hold them apart while she varnished her toenails and let them dry. I'd never set eyes on such things before.

Every night before bed, she would sit at the dressing table and put dabs of moisturising cream on her forehead and face then rub it in. I used to watch and tell her she didn't need to do it, her skin was nice anyway. 'If I want my skin to stay nice,' she would say, 'this is what I have to do.'

Something else I had never seen or heard of. Before cleaning her teeth she would pull out a bit of string from a small plastic container and run it between her teeth. Floss, she said, increasing my vocabulary by one. You don't have to use it on all your teeth, she said, just the ones you want to keep.

I tell you all this to demonstrate that her personal care had always been meticulous, her standards of hygiene the very highest.

'You keep telling me I'm beautiful, which embarrasses me,' she said to me more than once. 'Well, if I am, it's only because I do all this.' The truth, of course, was exactly the opposite. She was already beautiful: 'all this' was just maintenance.

Suchet's rule on female beauty: a truly beautiful woman is truly beautiful at six o'clock in the morning.

✳ ✳ ✳ ✳

Bon has taken a dislike to green vegetables, especially ones with soft leaves. Weird, from someone who has always been extremely aware of healthy food, and careful to make sure I had my daily intake of green vegetables. I emptied a pre-packed salad box onto her plate and mine. Before beginning to eat, Bon carefully picked the soft green leaves out of her salad with her fingers and laid them on the side of the plate. I watched in growing frustration. She had her fork in her left hand, and was picking out the leaves with her right. Her knife lay untouched. She was getting tomato dressing over her fingers, and I watched as she kept moving her fingers perilously close to her white cashmere cardigan.

I tried to say nothing. I ate. I felt a tightness across my chest. Finally I could bear it no longer. In as measured a voice as I could manage – though there was a tremor and false jollity to it – I said use your knife, darling, use your knife. That way your fingers will stay clean. I know, she said irritably, you don't have to tell me. She picked up her knife, put it down, and continued removing the dressing-covered leaves with her fingers. I reached for her knife and put it in her hand. She banged it down. I reached across again and removed the leaves from her plate onto mine. She began to eat, the tiniest mouthfuls, at a rate of about one a minute.

The tightness in my chest intensified. I tried to ignore her. After each small mouthful, she put her fork back down as if she had finished. It was tempting to take her plate away, but I had to make sure she ate more. Finally, she picked up her fork again, eating a tiny amount each time.

I continued eating, but found I was breathing in short shallow breaths. I felt as if my lungs were full of cement. I wanted to scream, shout, cry out, bang my head on the table. I dug my fingernails into the fleshy part of my arm until it hurt. That calmed me for a moment. But the silent saga continued: small piece of food to the mouth, tomato-covered fingers stroking white cardigan. I dug my nails into my forehead until the tears came. Then I remembered I was doing a Beethoven talk in a couple of days' time. Shit, the marks will show.

My obvious frustration simply compounded her confusion. Soon it was clear she didn't know whether to use her fork or knife, put them down on the table or plate, eat or drink. By reacting the way I was, I was simply making things worse. Finally she got up angrily from the table and said she needed to go to the toilet. She left the kitchen and headed down the corridor, missing the bathroom, to the bedroom. I went running after her. I couldn't risk an accident. You said you needed to go to the loo. I do, she said. Come on, I'll take you. She let me lead her to the bathroom. But it was a false alarm – only the five-thousandth false alarm of the morning.

By the time I sat down to watch the Grand Prix on television, I felt on the verge of a heart attack. Time to punch the living daylights out of a cushion. But even that is difficult. She picks up my frustration and anger, and it only adds to her confusion. When I had calmed down a bit – halfway or so through the race – I remembered how one woman had written to me telling me about her husband's dementia, and how every time she put a plate of food in front of him, he got up and put the plate in the airing cupboard. I've got it easy.

I am becoming more and more concerned. It is a month or so since Krakow, and things are sliding markedly. I don't know what to do about it. At the back of my mind lurks the one thought every carer dreads having to confront. The trip to Poland was, as I have said, horrendous, but the sole time Bon seemed comfortable was when we spent one night in a hotel in Radomsko. I was dreading it, because it was only hours after my personal little trauma. Also, a strange room. How would Bon cope, and what if I was taken ill and couldn't watch out for her?

They gave us their biggest room, but the bathroom was just three steps from the side of the bed on which Bon slept. I made sure the bathroom door was open and a dim light on when we went to sleep. I slept the sleep of the (nearly) dead, and heard practically nothing till about nine o'clock the next morning. I say practically, because I was aware in my sleep of Bon getting up and going into the bathroom, but did not have the strength to get out of bed. In fact, everything went like clockwork. When I mentioned it to her in the morning, she beamed from ear to ear, proud of her triumph and pleased at my satisfaction.

It is the fact that she was happy that weighs most on me now a month on as I run it through my mind again. Would it be kinder to her to be somewhere like that permanently, somewhere with her own bathroom just feet from her bed? My fingers have even half frozen above the computer keys as I write this. How can I even be contemplating it? And is the truth that it would make life easier for me, and that is why I am allowing myself to contemplate it? G is for Guilt.

We go to France a week from now for two-and-a-half weeks. For the first week, we will be without Monika. After Poland, I am dreading it. How will Bon cope in the house? How will *I* cope in the house? I think this trip might take the awful, but sooner or later inevitable, decision out of my hands.

Last weekend, I went up to Scotland for a long weekend reunion with three old university friends. We last did it two years ago. Then there were four wives, this time only three. I missed Bon, but I enjoyed every moment. I was able to move at my own pace, not all the time looking out for her. My friends took it upon themselves to relax me. When I arrived, they said I looked shattered. When I left, they said I had shed years. G-word, welcome again.

* * * *

It is morning now and last night was better. The early morning wandering did not happen. Could I dare hope for an improvement? No. I can hear Monika cajoling Bon to get dressed. Bon is raising her voice, swearing. Bonnie? Swearing? That's not my Bonnie, it simply is not her. I decide to intervene. I enter the bedroom and say sharply, 'Darling, why are you being so uncooperative?' She looks like a guilty schoolgirl and mutters, 'I am not being uncooperative.' 'Monika, leave her as she is, why struggle? Just leave her as she is.' Bon says yes and manages a half smile. 'But she is in her nightie,' Monika says. 'That's fine,' I say, 'we're not going out today, it's pouring with rain, she can stay as she is.'

Bonnie seems genuinely relieved, and we all calm down. As I write this, she is pacing the corridor in a pair of black slacks, her nightie, a long cardigan, the sun hat we bought in Cape Town, and some furry leather slippers I bought her in Krakow, which make an amazing squeak when she walks. She will stay like that all day. Why not? Path of least resistance. It makes me think the unthinkable once again.

* * * *

I long ago recognised the fundamental difference between men and women. It is all to do with how they take off a pullover. Watch a man take off a pullover. He reaches down his back with his hands, yanks it over his head, making a mess of his hair if he's got any, knocking his glasses off if he's wearing any, flailing his arms, knocking out anyone standing close on either side, ending up wondering if it was really worth it in the first place.

Now watch a woman perform the same manoeuvre. She reaches down to the front of the pullover, gently raises it over her contours, then – the crucial part – *crosses her arms* and lifts it gracefully over her head. Once clear of her head, she extricates one arm and then the other, and the pullover is removed. The whole operation has been performed with elegance and minimal usage of space. Her hair has stayed intact and no one has been injured.

I mention this because Bonnie, I discovered within hours of introducing her to my bedsit in DC, was an Olympic gold medallist in the pullover-removing event, a world champion. I remember to this day watching her remove her favourite pink cashmere cardigan outside a church in Austria on one of our Beethoven research trips. It was poetic elegance.

But she doesn't do it any more. Over the last few months, she has complained of a pain in her left shoulder. It is quite severe. It makes removing any item of clothing difficult, particularly long ones such as nightdresses. Undoubtedly this contributes to her reluctance to get dressed and undressed.

At first I was bewildered, but then I noticed something quite extraordinary. When removing a pullover, or any piece of clothing that needs to go over her head, instead of performing that wonderful manoeuvre that gave me such easy pleasure, she lifts the pullover, or whatever, over the *front* of her head and down to the back of her neck. This leaves the pullover stretched severely across her upper back. She is then stuck. I am now alert to this, and ease the pullover gently over one shoulder, then the other, and she is able to extricate her arms. With it finally off, she lets out a large gasp of relief, as if she has just been through a trauma, which in a way she has.

This has been going on for some time, since before she complained of the pain in her shoulder. I reckon that she must have been taking off a pullover in this new, bizarre way, become stuck, wriggled and strained to extricate herself, and pulled a muscle in her shoulder. Ever since, taking anything off over her head is traumatic.

There is a solution. As long as I am there, I can ease it forward over her head for her. I stand in front of her and tell her to put her hands on my shoulders. I then ease the pullover, or nightie, up over her head and towards me. She hates it, utterly hates it. I get it off as quickly as I can, but what I cannot avoid is the pullover or nightie messing up her hair. 'Look what you have done,' she shouts at me, tearing at her hair. 'You have made me look like a witch.'

It happened the other day with that same pink cashmere cardigan, and it hurt me to the pit of my stomach. I went off into another room and had a little cry. Dementia alters behaviour in all sorts of dramatic and distressing ways, but sometimes it is the little pleasures that are gone that hurt the most.

The usual difficult start to the day. Up at 6-ish, and a nice successful visit to the bathroom. But back to bed? Oh dear me, no. Compare this to how it once was. I said Bonnie was a gold medal pullover remover, but together for many years we were Olympic champion huggers. From day one in that Washington bedsit, we discovered the joy of a good hug. We would fall asleep hugging, and if we woke the next morning on opposite sides of the bed we would soon put it right. No matter what the day held, how early we had to be up, there was always time for a hug. No words, just wrapped up in each other. We fitted, we just fitted, from our lips to our toes. Bon summed it up one night early on in a single word. 'Skin,' she said. 'I need skin.'

I don't really know when it stopped, but I became aware that it made her feel a little uncomfortable, as if she was not entirely sure what was going on. I didn't try to explain, I just changed my behaviour and marked it down as another small victory for dementia.

So, on this particular morning, up she gets and the walking begins. Squeak, squeak. I get up a couple of times to make sure it is only walking, and nothing more. I try to get back to sleep, but know it is useless. Come back to bed, darling. Yes, I will. Sit on edge of bed. Up and walking again. We used to love our long corridor – gives the flat length. One of her American relatives once stood at the end of it, looked down the length of the flat, and said, 'Which part's yours?' Now I wish we were back in our bedsit; it would be easier to manage.

Finally I surrender, knowing it'll mean a doze in the chair later. I write late into the night, after I have got Bon to bed. It's the only time I can realistically do it. The early mornings then follow. So I'm guaranteed to fall asleep in an armchair in the afternoon, just like a drunken old fool after a heavy lunch.

Into the bathroom to brush my teeth, and there is the evidence that she did in fact do more than just walk. I must have missed it. Means a bath later, and the struggle that involves. Sod it. Damn and bugger it. I take it out on the egg boiler electric switch. Careful, John, break that and you really are fucked.

I cheer myself up by wondering whether I should put an ad in my local newsagent's window: *Wanted, friendly female for early morning hug, 6.30–7.30. No other duties required (yet).*

We are off to France on Monday. Am I dreading it? Is the Pope a Catholic? Does night follow day?

I had it all worked out for the journey down to Tardan tomorrow. Light dinner at the pasta place across the road, then a bath. Early to bed, because we need to get up at 3am for the ridiculously early flight, clean clothes laid out ready. It was a glorious late May weekend, so a nice walk in the park and an ice-cream. All going fine, except in the lift going back up to our flat she happened to mentioned her trousers had got wet near her shoes.

I was on instant alert. I reached out to feel the critical area. She recoiled. I remembered the CCTV camera in the top corner of the lift. Got to the flat and yep, sure enough, soaked. Everything. I lost it. Meant a bath now, clothes into the washer, dried quickly, because I would need some of them for the early morning start. Knew she would react angrily to the bath. Practically tore the clothes off her – I wasn't going to take any nonsense – and threw them into the machine.

Put her roughly into the bath. She was distressed and confused, and I was aware that my behaviour was only making things worse. But I simply couldn't control myself. It was the thought of all the plans going out of the window, but also fear, dread, about the following morning. What if she needed the toilet at the airport? I couldn't go in with her. I wanted to die. Really I did.

Got her out of the bath. She was struggling to understand what I was doing, but I had to move at my own pace, i.e. quickly, and I was not taking any argument. I knew I had to get her into nightclothes and dress-ing gown, which meant not going across the road for dinner. But we only had eggs in the fridge. OK, boiled bloody eggs for dinner. I braced myself. We had an egg poacher. I had never used it, but I remember watching Bon use it in years gone by.

I cracked the eggs into the little holders, marvelling that practically all the yolk actually went where I intended. I put the heat on to boil the water in the pan. Minutes passed. Bon was pacing the corridor, in distress. I was cursing the cooker. The water was boiling. Why wouldn't the eggs cook? Lightbulb on in head. Put lid on. Bon was now in the kitchen, and I saw her smile at me. *Smile?* How could she do that, after what I had done to her? It's all down to you, John: be happy and she is happy. It really was quite possible she had already forgotten what had happened.

I thought about this for a few moments, lifted the lid, and the eggs were hard. Shit. Slammed toast into the toaster, warned Bon the eggs would be a bit hard. She laughed and said that's all right. When I dished them up minutes later, to my utter amazement, they were perfect.

While we were eating them, the tumble dryer bleeped. I took out her clothes. I had managed to shrink her all-time favourite long white cashmere cardigan to about half its size. Still wearable, I figured, just a rather snug fit.

Dinner took about 10 minutes and then we went to bed. I lay in bed cursing myself, thinking how much worse I had made everything. And there was still the journey tomorrow to come.

* * * *

I am now writing this in our French house, on the evening of our arrival. And guess what? Bon was good as gold on the journey down. She plodded along happily behind me, with no idea where I was leading her. At Stansted I took the precaution of getting just one cup of tea and giving her only a few sips. On arrival at Pau airport, I got her a hot chocolate, her favourite. I took my heart in my hands and asked her if she needed the loo – better to have a go, whatever happened, rather than have an accident. She said no, she was fine. I, on the other hand, was bursting, but said nothing. Safer. We drove to the house. Only after an hour or so did she go to the toilet on her own, and all was fine.

I wanted to hug her, kiss her, thank her, and I wanted to beat myself unconscious for my behaviour, my fear, my everything.

I am still on red alert, obviously. I am not opening a bottle of wine this evening. It has always been one of our great pleasures down here, sipping chilled wine on the terrace watching the sun go down. Not tonight, Josephine. She won't complain, I know that.

Upstairs and into our beautiful wood-panelled bedroom, once the dusty old attic where the hay was stacked to dry and the mice ran riot, into nightclothes with just mild protestations, and to bed.

At breakfast I struggle with a honey jar. I can't get the top off. I spin round three times, enter Superman mode, and try again. It will not shift.

She says, 'That is a very recalcitrant lid.' You could have knocked me down with a feather.

Minutes later. 'I think I need to use the toilet. Can you remind me where it is?' Yes, my love, I certainly can.

* * * *

It is going to take me not years to become a master chef, but aeons. In fact, a lifetime is not long enough. Boy, did I pay the price for my cack-handed attempts to cook the other night. Down in France, no microwaveable boxes to save me. I cooked steak and some frozen mushrooms and broccoli. I don't know what possessed me. Bon doesn't eat a lot of red meat, and she said in advance it wasn't one of her favourites.

I went ahead anyway. First disaster was, I thought the frozen veggies were microwaveable, but they were not. On the back of the packets there were pictures of steamers, saucepans and frying pans, but no picture of a lovely microwave. Sod it, I thought, I'll microwave them anyway.

I dished up undercooked meat and half-frozen vegetables. I cut up Bon's steak for her, but she just picked at it. She managed a couple of small pieces, and a few pieces of mushroom. I ended up feeling pretty ashamed. I should, indeed could, have done better.

The next morning, her digestive system took full revenge on my appalling cooking. It was everywhere. In her clothes, on the floor, every-where, and as she moved from foot to foot, it spread ever further. I am totally ashamed to say I completely lost my temper. *Why didn't you tell me? Why didn't you say something?* I was shouting. She looked stunned and bewildered, and I realised she was not fully aware of what had happened. I gripped her by the upper arms, digging my fingers into the soft flesh, wanting to hurt her. Isn't that reprehensible? I actually wanted to hurt my Bonnie. How can that have happened?

It was 48 hours ago now, and I am able to recount it rationally. At the time I lost all sense of reason, I was in total despair, and Bon was staring at me, her eyes wide and uncomprehending. *Stand still*, I yelled at her, *stand still, do not move. Stand still, do you hear?* And I dug my fingers in again. She said, 'You are going to kill me, and I don't want you to kill me.' She actually said that, and for several seconds I thought that might be the answer. 'Yes,' I said, 'I will kill both of us.' I really did think that would put an end to all our problems. Hers, and mine. We would leave this world together, just as I had always intended we would.

My fingers have frozen over the keyboard again. Did this happen? Yes, it did. As I led her reluctantly into the walk-in shower this morning, I saw a blue bruise on her upper arm. I caused that, I did that to my Bonnie. I do not deserve to live.

Forty-eight hours on, my throat is still sore, and my voice strangled, from my shrieking. Bon, I believe, doesn't remember any of it. It took me a long time to clean things up. Thank God for the washing machine, which churned for the next six hours, though I used too much detergent, which flooded the sewage pipe in the garden.

I have calmed down now, come to my senses, and all I have left is an overwhelming sense of shame. Last night, I cooked a half-decent meal. A bland piece of chicken, with the same vegetables, though this time I steamed the broccoli and fried the mushrooms. I still didn't get it right. The broccoli had bits of ice on it, and I cremated the mushrooms and scorched the frying pan. There's no excuse, I should have got it right.

We sat on the terrace in lovely warm temperatures to eat. But Bon's eating has now slowed right down. It took her more than 30 minutes to eat the small plate of food. Twice, I heated it all up in the microwave to make it more palatable. It's strange. She no longer picks up her knife and fork together. Fork plus finger, mostly, and after each tiny mouthful she puts the fork back down on the table alongside the knife, as if she has finished. I have learned to wait.

We didn't exchange a word as she slowly picked at her food. At one point, I actually drifted off into a doze. I looked around the terrace sadly, remembering the animated voices and laughter that had resonated down the years as we ate and drank in this very spot with family and friends. How different it is now. Lonely and sad.

At lunch today – a simple plate of ham and cheese – I took the obvious next step. As she sat there, staring at the food, occasionally moving a tiny amount to her mouth (I had long finished mine), I first cut up her ham, then fed it to her … or rather, put it on her fork and handed the fork to her. You don't have to do this, you know, she said smiling, but she didn't stop me. We had her plate finished within a minute.

Dinner was a better affair all round. I finally mastered the mushrooms. Bon ate everything, and in a normal amount of time. We settled down in front of the telly for the evening, and then it all went wrong.

Claudette, who with her husband Jean-Pierre sold us the house 20 years ago and who lives just up the road, came at around nine to say *bonsoir*. She pointed out that I had left the bathroom light on, above the toilet. I nodded and smiled. She understood. She and I sat in the *séjour*, chatting away in French. Mostly we talked about Bon. Claudette said she and Jean-Pierre could not believe how thin she had become, in her face. I pointed out that actually she had put on weight, having developed a taste for sweet food. While we chatted, Bon simply walked round and round and round.

After Claudette left, Bon came to sit with me and we watched telly. An hour later, bedtime. We walked into the kitchen and that's when I saw the first tell-tale signs. Tiny puddles. I walked further in, and then saw a trail of tiny puddles all around the small corridor, outside the bathroom, and across the large salon where the staircase is. Bon had walked around, simply letting it go, just feet away from the toilet, where the door was open and the light on. I gasped at the extent of it, but kept calm.

I leapt into action. I got Bon into the shower – she protested, but only mildly, and I ignored it – and her clothes into the washing machine. I got her into a clean nightie and upstairs into bed. Then I came down and mopped everywhere. Thank God for a tiled floor, which I knew would be dry by the morning. The biggest problem, and I knew it, was that she had come and sat with me to watch telly. Yep, sure enough, the armchair cushion was soaked. I sponged it down, but I know that is not enough. I don't know what to do about it.

Good night's sleep, and up this morning at six. In the following hour, five visits to the toilet, and one during breakfast. Nothing. I am on red alert. *Red alert.*

It cannot go on like this, it cannot. My Bonnie is losing the daily rhythm of life. She is confused and unhappy, and I am contributing to her unhappiness. I believe the French idyll, which began with so much excitement and expectation, and has lasted for 20 years, must soon be over.

* * * *

Monika arrived as planned and I knew the worst was over for me. We sat at the kitchen table while I briefed her about the last few days. Bonnie was doing her wandering, up and down the kitchen, into the *séjour* and back out again. She kept shooting me a look – it was a mixture of suspicion and mild anger, as if she suspected I was talking about her.

It turned into a baking hot day. Monika insisted we all drank lots of water. I gave her a knowing look. She brushed it aside. 'It is important not to get dehydrated,' she said.

Sure enough, a couple of hours later, the inevitable consequence. I went into panic mode, but Monika calmly mopped up, got the shower going, got out clean clothes. Why can't I handle these things properly? I feel useless, inadequate.

But it raised the whole summer issue again. Can we come down here for weeks on end, as planned? I simply don't know. I don't know what to do, what decision to make.

I am seeing Ian when we get back, and I am going to discuss it with him, raise the question, the dreaded unmentionable question. Full-time care. It sounds cruel, and I feel cruel even thinking about it. Sitting here writing about it, thinking about it, while all the time Bonnie is just walking around, Monika's sunglasses on, occasionally glancing at me, having not the slightest idea what is going through my mind.

Monika has just spotted Bon is wearing her sunglasses. She asks gently for them. Bon refuses. Monika says (rather cleverly), 'Here, I'll give you yours, you can give me mine.' No luck. Bon is adamant. Monika gives up.

Complete getting dressed crisis this morning. It has been getting more and more difficult. This morning, it was impossible. Would the nightie come off? It would not. I tried gently, several times. Monika tried. Resistance, argument, raised voices, even aggression. *(Bonnie? Aggressive?)* In the end, I made the decision to stop fighting. Ian has advised me, always the path of least resistance. 'Leave her,' I said. I showered and dressed, and as I write this, at almost 10 o'clock in the morning, Bon is walking round in her dressing gown and slippers.

I battered my head against it like a bull, but Monika thought round it. 'The problem is that the only things we ever discuss with her are going to the toilet and getting dressed and undressed. Remember when it was the glass of water obsession, when she would put five or six glasses of water on a tray? Or when it was the flushing the toilet obsession – dozens of times a day? Now it is the nightdress. So we must stop using the nightdress. Don't put it on her at night. Let her go to bed in her undies. It will make the morning so much easier.'

Good girl, Monika. I think again how much easier, and less distressing for Bon, it will be back in London, or, even, yes, that dreaded H-word again, a home.

We are coming to the end of this particular stay down in France – a little over two weeks, much shorter than usual, but I have a number of gigs – Beethoven and dementia – when we get back. I am still in two minds about the summer. We are due back down in six weeks. Should we come? We seem now to have developed a sort of routine. Not putting the nightie on last night worked an absolute treat. A bit reluctant to go into the shower this morning, but not bad. I handle that part of it. Out she comes, I help her dry, and as if by magic there is Monika with a clean set of clothes to help her dress. Went (almost) like clockwork this morning. She is now walking round the house while I tap tap, but she is happy.

Another development. She is eating almost normally. She finishes her plate at lunch and dinner. It takes a while, but she is eating better than I have seen for ages. Obviously it's to do with the fact that Monika is dishing up proper meals, instead of the rubbish I managed. But also it may have something to do with settling in down here. I really don't know.

Claudette popped round last night and sat with us on the terrace. Bon sat too, not wandering, smiling and happy, even though the entire conversation was about her, in French. Claudette pointed out Bon had picked up a bit of sun, and how well it made her look. It was true. She always looks better towards the end of a stay down here than at the beginning. So she is clearly deriving some benefit.

Right, decision made (for the moment, at any rate). We will come, the three of us, as planned in late July for two months (with a break in the middle for a family wedding). The first week or so will be traumatic, but then things should get easier as she settles down.

I love living in our little village, but the smallness of it makes gossip inevitable. We were in the local *épicerie* the other morning, buying bread and stuff, and Anne, who we know well, and who knows about Bon, greeted us warmly. When we got to the till with a load of stuff, I paid, packed the basket, and asked Bon if she would carry the apple tart (local speciality), which I had bought. 'Of course,' she said, putting out both hands so she could hold it flat. She then passed it Anne, who looked at me and smiled, indicating she understood, and gently guided Bon's hands to me. I thought then, I bet that'll be right round the village in no time. Hey ho. Never mind. There are worse things they could say.

* * * *

A week later to the day was the very worst morning of my life. I know I have said it before, but this time it really was the worst. We were back in London and I was tense from the moment we got up. At 10.30, a television producer was coming to see me to discuss making a documentary about Bonnie and me. I had lain in bed since Bon first got up around five, thinking about it. I didn't want TV cameras intruding into our lives (ironic, no?), but after all the publicity that followed my 'going public' I was not surprised there was interest.

There was something else. I had been contacted by an old colleague at ITN asking me to present a series of short programmes after *News at Ten* to commemorate the 40th anniversary of Apollo 11 and the first moon landing. I was, as with the TV documentary request but for different reasons, torn. My heart wanted more than anything to say yes. Back in the old building, the newsroom I had worked in for years, the studio where I had presented my last *News at Ten*, seeing old colleagues again. It was wonderful, and flattering to have been asked. My head said don't be a fool, it's five years since you left ITN, you've had your day, things have moved on, what if you make an idiot of yourself? My heart won. I was going in to begin work at three o'clock that afternoon.

I was making an early breakfast for us (yes, the egg-boiling machine again), Monika being in Poland at a family wedding. Bonnie was nowhere to be seen. 'Breakfast, darling,' I called out down the corridor. I went back to pour the cereal. Bonnie came into the kitchen. I smiled at her, she smiled back, then I saw the stain. I caught a momentary look of panic in her eyes. I walked back down the corridor, into the bedroom, and wanted to die. I wanted my heart to stop beating. My knees went weak and my stomach turned to lead. My initial thought was 'How on earth …?' My next thought was 'How am I going to deal with this?' It was like what happened in the bathroom in France, but ten times worse, a hundred times worse. The first thing I did was open the window, taking care where I stepped.

She walked into the room. I tried to control myself. 'You've had an accident.' 'Yes,' she said, with a small smile. 'Why didn't you say something?' I asked quietly, but menacingly. *'Why didn't you say something?'* I screamed at her. She turned and fled. I looked around. Clean up the bedroom, or clean up Bonnie? I knew cleaning up Bonnie was the priority, but I also knew she would protest like hell, and I wasn't sure I could stand that. I looked again at the bedroom floor. How to clean it up? I felt my breath quicken and my chest begin to hurt. I waited for my heart to stop. I *wanted* my heart to stop.

I went into the bathroom and got out disinfectant and a plastic bowl. But again I knew Bonnie was the priority. *'Come into the bathroom,'* I shouted. She came in, gingerly. I took off her dressing gown and threw it to the ground. 'I'll have to get you out of your nightie. It's filthy.' I looked at her challengingly, daring her to protest. I tore the nightie over her head, she stamped her feet and screamed. I lost my temper. I grabbed her by the arms, digging my fingers in, just as I had done in France. Panic shot into her eyes, she lashed her arms out, and I felt her nails slash down my cheeks. I caught my breath with pain. Her eyes stared at me. The same thought had gone through her mind as in France and she had done the most natural thing – she had defended herself. In a split second, I knew that her reaction was instinctive, that if I had not behaved so utterly appallingly – again – she would not have done what she had done. The fact remained that for the first time in our entire relationship, ever, Bonnie had been violent towards me, and it was my fault, *my fucking fault.*

She stood looking at me in horror, whether at what she had done or I had done, I couldn't tell. I put my hands to my cheeks. I felt the sticky warmth on my fingers. 'Look what you've done. You've drawn blood.' 'You scared me,' she said.

In an instant, I calmed down. She had brought me to my senses. 'Come on, let me get you into the bath,' I said softly. While she sat in the bath, I tackled the bedroom. It took me half an hour to clear things up. I got her out of the bath and she thanked me, she actually thanked me. The truly extraordinary thing is that, by the time we had finished breakfast, she had forgotten about the whole thing. Dementia, bloody hell.

I rang the television producer, told her I was having to deal with a somewhat unexpected problem. She was great. Just call me whenever you're ready, she said. I put some sticky plaster on the scratches, and when she came up to the flat an hour or so later I sat, elbows on the table, hands covering my cheeks, hoping she wouldn't notice (although she can't have failed to notice the overwhelming aroma of Dettol, which lasted for weeks). In the afternoon I dressed in suit and tie, pulled my shirt cuffs down just enough so my discreet gold cufflinks peeked out, and went into ITN. Nobody said anything about my dodgy face, but they wouldn't, would they? It was with some relief that I sat in the makeup chair.

I can't remember at what point in the day I made the connection, but it was 29th June, our 24th wedding anniversary.

Flashback to 29th June 1995, our 10th wedding anniversary. I booked a table for dinner at a restaurant run by a new breed of masterchef. I chose it because this one happened to be French, happened to have been born and raised in Gascony, and was cooking Gascon food in London. The meal was spectacular, as was the bill. Didn't matter. Not for the first, or even thousandth, time we talked about the past, marvelling at how insurmountable obstacles had been overcome, impossible dreams had been realised. We were man and wife, we lived in an elegant apartment in London and an adorable farmhouse in Gascony. I reminded her I was a mere poodle and she threw her head back and laughed at the memory of another dinner.

I chose my moment well. Over a glass of Sauternes (grapes grown about an hour from Tardan, I reminded her), I took a small box out of my pocket. She gasped at the sight of a delicate brooch, two lovebirds in blue and green, on a gold perch, wings entwined. I didn't have to say anything.

Another glass of Sauternes, she opened her handbag and took out a small box. A beautiful pair of discreet gold cufflinks. Yes, the same cufflinks I wore on that day 14 years later for the Apollo 11 programmes. The watch I was still wearing, the pen I still used – all bought for me by Bonnie.

I finished the ITN job and flew straight to Atlanta to see my son Rory, who had been working for CNN but was shortly to move to Moscow where he had landed a job as reporter/presenter for Russia Today, Russia's English-language news channel. I got an e-mail from Monika while I was there. There had been a repeat of what had happened with me, this time in the sitting room. Cream carpet, not good. My shoulders literally sagged as I read her account. But she had handled it a thousand times better than me, with no trauma. The next day a much better e-mail. All was fine.

When I got back and walked into the flat, Bonnie greeted me with the broadest smile I had seen for a long time. 'There you are,' she said excitedly, ' I haven't seen you for ages.' It was lovely to hear, but as I walked towards her I could see that there was no recognition in her eyes, or that was how it seemed. I put my arms round her. She allowed me to, but barely reciprocated. We sat in our usual chairs in the sitting room. I marvelled at the good job Monika had done on the carpet, compared to my botched attempt in the bedroom.

I looked at Bon, and was overwhelmed with a desire to know if she really recognised me. 'Come on,' I said enthusiastically, 'make me really happy. Tell me my name.' She threw her head back and laughed. 'I know who you are,' she said, 'don't be silly.' 'Of course you do, I know you do,' I said. A pause, and then, 'Come on, tell me my name.' She wagged her finger at me, still smiling, 'I'll tell you your name when you tell me yours.' I had been away for five days.

We interrupt this scintillating and laugh-a-minute narrative to bring you breaking news. The distinguished British conductor and Verdi specialist Sir Edward Downes and his wife of 54 years have died together at the clinic in Zurich run by the assisted suicide group Dignitas.

Let us pause for a moment to look at that in a little more detail. Sir Edward, universally known as Ted, was 85 years of age, going blind and losing his hearing. He knew he would not conduct again. His wife Joan was recently diagnosed with inoperable cancer of the liver and pancreas.

According to their two children, they died 'peacefully and under circumstances of their own choosing'. They wanted to be next to each other when they died, their son said, and they held hands across the beds.

Reading the details, I realised that deep in the recesses of my impossibly romantic mind, that was the kind of thing I'd had in mind for Bonnie and me. Ideally it would have been brought about by extreme old age rather than illness, and in our own bed rather than anywhere else, but imagine – lying alongside each other at the moment of your choosing. How could you better that? I salute you, Sir Ted.

Before going to the States, I braced myself and discussed full-time care with Ian. He said Bonnie was without doubt ready. 'She needs professional care,' he said, 'more than you or Monika are able to give.' I argued with him. My main concern was that I was considering this purely for my own benefit, to make my life easier. 'That is half true,' Ian said. 'The timing needs to be right for both of you, not just Bonnie. It is for your benefit as well as hers. You have your life to consider. The strain of caring can kill.' He let his words hang in the air. 'Another thing,' he went on, 'it's important to put someone with dementia into full-time care when they are still able to do a lot of things, when they are not too far down the road. If you wait too long, the moment will come when you have to act, the decision is taken out of your hands, but then it will be crisis management, and that is the worst thing that can happen. The staff in the care home don't know the person coming in, the person doesn't know them, no preparations have been made. Believe me, John, hard and painful though it may be for you to accept this, in my view Bonnie is absolutely ready to go into full-time care.'

I discussed it with Bon's sons, Alec and H. I don't know why, but I expected to receive a lot of grief from them. *Our mother, the woman you say you love, yet you are considering putting her into a home?* In the event, they both said they completely understood, and they would support me if that was the decision I made. They reminded me it was now more than three years since the diagnosis, that they had lived with the knowledge of their mum's illness for a long time, and from some of the things I had told them could barely begin to imagine what I was going through. H said that if I were going to look at places, he would like to come too. I was relieved. I didn't want to have to make the decision alone.

I returned from the States, and on an afternoon in early July 2009, H and I went to see a care home in Berkshire. I was tired from the overnight flight, and wasn't looking forward to the inevitable emotion this would entail. He met me at the station and we drove to the home, barely speaking, both bracing ourselves. In the event, it was far, far worse than we had been expecting.

A group of very elderly people in their eighties and nineties sitting in a room playing bingo. Puddles of spilled drinks on the floor. Small bedrooms. Is this what all care homes are like? We barely exchanged glances as we were shown round. In the car outside, we looked at each other. We were both trying to suppress tears. My son Damian had told me his grannie-in-law had recently moved into a care home in Surrey that was truly lovely, like a hotel. It was one of a chain called Sundial. In the car we looked it up, and there was a branch just 10 minutes from where we were. We decided to have a quick look – reluctantly, because neither of us wanted to go through that experience again.

Even as we drove up to it, we could tell it was different. It actually looked like a country hotel. We walked in unannounced, were quickly swept up by the manageress, who spent the next hour showing us around. The atmosphere was friendly, the rooms truly attractive. In the car afterwards, H said to me he would be happy for his mum to be there. Thank goodness we had bothered to go and look.

I got home later than I had promised. Bon once again smiled broadly to see me. If she had only known how I had spent my afternoon. I couldn't hold back the tears.

✳ ✳ ✳ ✳

A psychiatrist from Westminster NHS has just been to assess Bonnie. He asked her point blank how she was. She recoiled slightly and said, 'I'm fine, thank you.' He said, 'And what have you been doing today?' 'Not much,' she said, 'what about you?' It was his turn to recoil slightly. 'I'm trying to assess how you are,' he said, making me want to sink my head in my hands. 'I'm fine,' Bon said slightly aggressively. 'How are you?' I wanted to cheer for her. 'That's fine,' he said, looking at me and gesturing that we should move into another room to talk. 'I'm just going to have a talk with your husband,' he said. No surprise that a look of suspicion clouded her face. She knew we weren't going to discuss football.

In the dining room, he said he had never met any person with dementia as calm and relaxed as Bonnie. I was surprised at first, not least because the whole conversation had consisted of no more than a few sentences, but that fitted with her character. I told her years ago that the most violent thing she ever did was sneeze. 'Do you think that means she's not ready to go into full-time residential care?' I asked hopefully. He shook his head. 'The opposite,' he said. 'Tell me, when you are down in France, does she ask about the flat?' 'No.' 'When you are here in the flat, does she ask about France?' 'No.' 'Well, all this implies she would settle well into a home.' That really pulled me up short.

Bonnie has been very confused today. She hasn't followed what I have said, and when she has responded it hasn't made sense. For a long period this afternoon, while I sat watching television, she walked up and down the corridor. This is not her usual behaviour – if I sit in front of the telly, she usually does too. It was a chill July day, and her walking made her shiver. I had a fan heater on in the sitting room. Several times I gently implored her to come and sit down in the warmth. Each time she said yes, and continued her wandering. But she was not in poor spirits. When she saw me, her face would break into a smile. But I was concerned nonetheless.

Next day, and it turns out to be a day full of emotion. It began with a visit to our GP for a sort of pre-summer check-in, to get repeat prescriptions for the planned two months down in France. Our GP, of course, knows all about Bon, and has been wonderful with advice and comfort for me. This morning we sat with her. Bon smiled, responding with a little chit-chat to the GP's questions. It was a slightly surreal conversation. 'Hello, Bonnie, how are you?' 'I'm fine, how are you?' 'I'm fine too.

I haven't seen you for a long time.' 'Don't be silly. I see you all the time.' 'Of course. Well, it's good to see you again.' 'Yes, I haven't seen you for ages.' And so on.

I launched into a kind of weird coded conversation about the care home H and I had found. I said *hotel* instead of *home*. I said we were planning to go away probably in the autumn to this place, gesturing to Bonnie with my head. The GP smiled knowingly. I said it was a really nice place. Bon nodded agreement with everything I said. It's a technique she uses to give the impression she is following the conversation. I decided to be bold. 'What do you think of the timing?' I asked. 'Absolutely, definitely,' said the GP, 'it is the right decision, for both of you.'

I said, sort of *sotto voce*, 'There's this wretched guilt demon on my shoulder,' and I tapped my shoulder. The GP flicked her fingers on her shoulder. 'Get rid of that, totally,' she said, continuing to flick. Bon registered nothing. 'And make an appointment to come and see me. Before. You will have reactions you won't expect. I can help you.' I nodded my thanks. Bon nodded too.

Back home, I weighed up the advice. Three people, all specialists, had now made the same recommendation. There was a fourth, too. As a direct result of all the publicity after I went public about Bon back in February, Ian had been promoted within the charity to reorganise and run the dementia helpline. I was to be given a new Admiral Nurse, Alison. She had already sat in on sessions I had had with Ian, and she had met Bonnie too. Although pointing out she was new to my 'case', as it were, from everything she had seen and heard, she concurred with Ian that Bon was ready for full-time care. So, Admiral Nurses Ian and Alison, the psychiatrist, and now our GP. All said they were sure not just that Bonnie was ready for full-time care, but that she and I would both actually benefit from it.

I sat with Bonnie in front of the telly for the rest of the day. I wanted to be with her. I knew if I sat, she would sit. If I tried to write, or do any other kind of work, she would get up and pace. I just wanted her calm peaceful company. I also needed mindless TV programmes to help my mind wander.

At around six o'clock, performing the task as swiftly as I could, I went to the computer and wrote an e-mail to Sundial, booking Bon in for a six-week trial period beginning in early October, when I am busy with dementia conferences. Before that, two months in France. At least, that's the plan. Bon wandered in and out of the dining room, watching me type, with no idea at all of what I was doing. I was on the brink of tears the whole time.

I dished up a microwave dinner and tears were brimming in my eyes. Bonnie, thankfully, did not notice. Later in the evening, after *News at Ten*, there I was on the small screen: 16th July 2009, 40 years to the day since Apollo 11 blasted off. Bon sat watching without reacting. No comment at all. There was only one medium close-up. I was pleased to see the make-up artist had done a good job. No sign at all of the trauma that had unfolded at home. How thoroughly professional I looked. I sat watching myself as if I were looking at some entirely different creature. On screen, the television presenter with decades of experience, able to cope with anything they threw at him. In the armchair, watching him, an emotional wreck with tears pricking at the back of his eyes and a sodden tissue in his hand.

I got Bon to bed, and here I am writing about it. I have just committed my darling Bonnie, the love of my life, to a care home, and she knows nothing about it, nothing at all. I can't flick the guilt demon off my shoulder, I can't, he's too strong. If I'm not careful, he will destroy me.

I am going out to Sundial today to meet the Executive Director and the Director of Community Relations (sounds a bit formal) to discuss Bonnie's needs and choose a room for October. I must admit that when I got up this morning, knowing there would be trauma with the clean-up when it came to getting dressed, I began to think of the stay in the home with a slight feeling of relief. How will I feel after two months in France? It makes me smile a little to think of my utter wretchedness in making the decision, and the fact that now I am looking forward to it just very, very slightly. *Get off my shoulder, little guilt demon.*

Contemplating the grimness of the day ahead, the emotion of going out to the home, I sat in the sitting room with Bon. We both stared silently into space.

'Waiting for Godot,' she said, turning to me. Another knock-me-down-with-a-feather moment.

* * * *

The visit to Sundial was gruelling. Talking about Bonnie, about our idyllic relationship, explaining her decline … I rabbitted on. It was plug-pulled-out syndrome. They were good listeners. We went upstairs to the dementia unit. Much, much nicer than that makes it sound. It's called Reminiscence, which is actually rather evocative. They showed me the only available room. It was small but nice, with a spectacular view of greenery. In the bathroom, there was a walk-in shower, which was good.

I thought of the countless hotel rooms Bon and I have walked into over the years, the double beds we have thrown ourselves onto, the champagne we have uncorked. Now I was looking at an empty room – to be furnished by me so it is familiar to Bon – in which Bon might well spend (how can I bring myself to write this) the rest of her life.

The woman in charge of Reminiscence is an irrepressibly cheerful and smiley woman named Louise. Standing in the empty room, I was pouring out my woes, saying that since going public about Bonnie I seemed to have become the public face of dementia, a spokesman for carers, I was having to learn an awful lot awfully fast, and it was not exactly the role I had envisaged for my retirement.

Louise nodded – that smile never leaving her face for even a second – saying she knew what I meant. She said she had a young son with severe Down's Syndrome. He had trouble with his jaw muscles, so had great difficulty eating and drinking. The specialists had told Louise he would probably not live beyond 30, and was likely to develop severe dementia in his final years. 'So I found myself suddenly having to learn about Down's,' Louise said. 'It wasn't what I wanted, but I thought, well, this has happened, I had better find out as much about it as I can.' I felt about two feet tall.

As a result of the visit, I have curtailed our summer plans in France. Sundial want to do a lot of research on Bon, Louise wants to come with a colleague to meet her, assess her, before she goes in. I had intended Bon going in during the swift week in October between coming back from France and me doing the dementia conferences. But I realised as we spoke that I was simply trying to sandwich everything in, putting me and everyone else under pressure. And if I felt under pressure, I knew Bon would instinctively inherit the tension from me.

I made a decision there and then. We go to France as planned next Monday. We stay for the whole of August. Once back, I set everything in motion for Sundial, and Bon moves in on 15th September. It means this will be the last trip together to Tardan, the house we bought 20 years ago for our retirement. That dream is over – but I have known that really for the last two years. It is just that the moment has come now, rather than later.

I returned from Sundial late afternoon, exhausted emotionally and physically. I had just booked my Bonnie into a home. How could I have done that? *How? How?* Bon welcomed me back into the flat. She knew nothing, absolutely nothing of what I had been doing. I walked into the dining room and unpacked my briefcase. I had been given a huge folder to fill in for Sundial.

I heard Bon in the bathroom, and the gentle tinkle which meant she was spending a penny. I hurried in to offer the paper. I saw immediately that while her slacks were round her ankles, she had not taken her undies down. Small puddles were forming on the floor. She looked up at me, with panic in her eyes at how I might react.

I smiled. Yes, I surprised myself and smiled. 'Never mind,' I said breezily. 'Come on, I'll help you clean up. Shall I give you a nice bath?' I asked, still smiling. 'Yes,' she said, returning my smile. I got her undressed and she didn't complain. I was still smiling, and therefore so was she. 'Anyway,' I said, 'I like getting you undressed for the bath. Gives me a chance to see your boobs.' She roared with laughter. The bath went the best it had ever gone.

I was happy because her incontinence was final proof to me that she was ready for full-time care. It was what I needed to set my mind at rest, flick the guilt demon from my shoulder. It was as if she was saying to me, 'Don't worry, my darling, you're doing the right thing, you are doing what is best for me.'

So I am telling myself.

I woke up at four in the morning after the Sundial decision, overwhelmed at what I was doing. I lay there thinking, unable to get to sleep, and in the clarity of the small hours I worked out some sort of logic to it all. Bonnie is now two people. There is the Bonnie I loved, who is gone, and there is the Bonnie who is still here with me. They are two different Bonnies. The one I am now putting into a home is the Bonnie who is still here with me, not the other one. Therefore I must not think I am doing this to the Bonnie I fell in love with, with whom I lived in such intimate intensity for all those years, with whom I shared every aspect of my life. I am doing it to the Bonnie who is here with me now, who had that accident on the toilet, who is walking up and down the corridor of our flat as I sit here writing this, who actually *needs* full-time care and will benefit from it.

Chapter 13

So here we are in France for what will be the last visit together. For 20 years, the journey down has been a mixture of laughter and excitement. This time, it was like a dead weight on my shoulders. When we arrived, Bonnie showed no recognition, and soon took up her walking circuit. Monika bustled around, doing all the things Bonnie used to do, finally knocking up a good dinner. And still Bon walked.

There is a new obsession. Bonnie is always cold. That in itself is not particularly new. For years I have joked with her about how her hands and feet are always cold, even if the rest of her is warm and the weather is warm too. She told me years ago it was down to low blood pressure, and that many a doctor had told her she should be grateful, low blood pressure was a good thing. Cold extremities were a small price to pay. Anyway, I have exactly the opposite problem. I am always too warm, so it has never been an arduous – or unenjoyable – task to warm her up.

But in the last few months it has become a visibly distressing problem. She actually shivers, hunching her shoulders and clutching her hands in front of her. I check, and unbelievably her hands are not all that cold, certainly not as cold as they used to be. And she doesn't seem unduly worried. Although shivering, teeth chattering, she will smile and say I'm fine, I'm fine. I put fan heaters on, dress her in more layers, which works for a short while and then she says she is too hot.

I found myself looking forward to France in August, if for no other reason than that she should not feel uncomfortably cold. But it hasn't worked out that way.

This morning, Morning Number One, a disastrous attempt to get Bon dressed. I gave up and told Monika not to try, for fear of upsetting her more. After breakfast she resumed her walking, the well-established circuit of *séjour* kitchen *séjour* kitchen, shivering in her dressing gown, despite wonderful sunshine flooding into the house. Monika had the good idea of bringing her clothes down to the bathroom, which was nice and warm with the towel radiator on. I could hear Bon objecting. Monika was pleading gently, warning that she would have to come and get me if Bon didn't comply. Bon just wouldn't have it. I went into the bathroom. Bon was standing in her nightie, a defiant look on her face. I said, 'Enough. Stop. No fighting, Monika. Darling, put your dressing gown back on. Stay exactly as you are.' She let me help her put it back on. Now she is doing her circuit again, shivering in her dressing gown.

We have a month of this ahead of us.

She stayed in her dressing gown and nightie all day. In the evening I decided to go round to say hello to Jean-Pierre and Claudette. It is something we traditionally do at the beginning of each visit. I couldn't take Bon, because she was still in her dressing gown, so I went alone. Just a short drive. I stood with them and we talked about Bon. I told them of my decision to put her into a home. They said it was absolutely the right decision, and it would do me as much good as her. She won't know, said Claudette dogmatically, she will have no idea. I hope she is right. I told them of the struggle to get Bon showered this morning, and how I had given up after three attempts. Claudette said, in her direct way, 'Scold her'. I couldn't help looking a bit shocked. It was the direct opposite of all the advice I have been given. But it's a thought.

I finally made my excuses and left them. I got back to the house, where Monika was preparing dinner. Her face was a mask of horror, she was flushed and breathless. She blurted out, 'You will not believe what happened. When you left, Bonnie followed you.' She explained that Raymonde, our neighbour, had come hurrying over and gesticulated, saying 'Bonnie! Bonnie!' and pointing out to the road. She said she went running out, but Bonnie was nowhere to be seen in our cul de sac. She ran to the end of it, and there was Bonnie, in the middle of the main road, in her nightie and dressing gown, halfway to Jean-Pierre and Claudette's.

I listened in utter horror. Bon has never done that before. She heard Monika explaining what had happened, but just smiled and said nothing. I honestly think she had already forgotten.

I thought about it in bed, and in a way I felt sort of comforted that it had happened. It was yet another sign that I had made the right decision. It seems as if I am constantly looking for more evidence that the time is right, as if I don't trust my instincts, despite all the advice I am receiving. That's it, I suppose – I really don't trust my instincts. What if she doesn't settle into Sundial at all? What if it's a total disaster? I fell asleep totally depressed.

Woke up this morning feeling a lot better. Amazing what screeching birds and a blast of sunshine through the windows can do. After breakfast, the shower issue again. Bonnie was shivering in her dressing gown, and it had been two days since she'd had a good wash, so it had to happen. I said shower time and she said fine. Got her into the bathroom and all the old problems. Monika said, 'Be angry.' OK, Claudette first, now Monika. Who am I to disagree? Emboldened, I got angry. Bonnie responded instantly, muttering curses, but doing what she was told. Into the shower, Monika took over, and she loved it. The new walk-in shower I've had put in is ideal, no hauling in and out of a bath, soaping is easy. It's what they have at Sundial too, which is good.

Bon is now dressed, warm, resuming her walking circuit. We have done it. But I can scarcely believe I scolded my darling Bonnie. If you had ever told me in those golden years I would do that, I would have told you that you were mad. I once said to Bonnie, after we had been together for around 20 years, 'I think we have had two rows.' 'Have we?' she asked. 'When?'

* * * *

Bonnie is a great gardener. I know there are men gardeners prancing around on television, just like men chefs, but I think it is a woman thing. Women instinctively like cooking and instinctively like gardening, whereas men *may* like them. I don't, as it happens.

Given that Bonnie loves gardening so much, you can see what I was depriving her of by asking her to live with me in a flat in London. Not even a windowbox. Equally, you can see what I was offering her with our tumbledown French farmhouse. An acre of garden, no less, for her to do as she liked with. True, she said to me quite early on, 'When I told you I wanted a garden, I didn't expect you to give me one 600 miles away, but that's fine, I'm not complaining.'

She set about the garden in Tardan with relish. I learned of varieties of trees I had never heard of, learned that there are other types of flower apart from tulips, daffodils and roses (the only ones I could identify), and struggled to understand why it is that simply watering plants is not enough, you have to be careful not to *over*-water them. Sounded bizarre, but I trusted her. She also cautioned me that much as I might long for the sun to tan my manly torso, if there was too much of it the garden would need extra watering. Patiently, without really knowing what I was doing, I spent many an hour directing a hosepipe towards some kind of plant or other, watering away from the roots for the trees (something about encouraging them to spread out to find the water – weird), and managing to drown almost as many flowering shrubs as I kept alive.

'You city boy,' she used to say, but there was laughter in her voice.

Together we planted shrubs along the end of the terrace. She said they would grow to form a low hedge, giving us privacy. They did, and then she used to take advantage of that to sunbathe in a swimsuit on the lounger, the timer set to exactly 10 minutes for front and back, so as not to burn her delicate skin. On many an occasion, I would encourage her to take even more advantage of the privacy that hedge afforded, and I'd lie on the lounger alongside her relishing the sight of her. 'You're embarrassing me,' she would say quietly. That was always my cue to kiss her and gently move her swimsuit back into place.

That hedge is there now, today, fully grown. 'Look darling, remember how we planted that hedge together in the sweltering heat?' She smiles and nods.

* * * *

Bonnie has started walking bent to the side at the hip, not far off 45°. At one point, she almost keeled over. I pointed it out to her, and she couldn't see that anything was wrong. Her face looked terribly confused. I asked her if she was in pain and she said no.

I became so worried I even checked the emergency number to call if we should need an ambulance, and I e-mailed my Admiral Nurse Alison to ask her what she thought. Then, after a couple of hours, it stopped as suddenly as it started. It's the next morning now, and she's fine. Confused, certainly, but no worse than usual, and no obvious list when she walks.

Alison e-mailed back, wondering whether Bonnie has had a mini-stroke. That made me gasp out loud. It's not just the walking; her confusion is so much worse. I can see her straining to comprehend what is going on. Could she have had a mini-stroke? I remember my Dad in his final years moving his arm in a strange way, bent back at the elbow as if constantly trying to push something out of the way. I was intolerant of it, then a geriatrician suggested it was the result of a small stroke.

I was covered in guilt, and now I feel the same way again. The more I consider it, the more I wonder if this is not what has happened to my darling Bonnie. I will be kinder to you, my love, more tolerant, I really will. If that is what has happened, you poor, poor darling. I know what this can mean. Once you've had one stroke, you're more likely to have more, like Dad did. God.

* * * *

Bonnie stands at the kitchen door, staring out into the garden. There is a searching look on her face, her eyes slightly screwed closed, her mouth tense and half open. I remember the same in my dad's face. She also has a new physical habit, constantly reaching back with her right hand to adjust her slacks and underwear. I mean constantly. Every five seconds, while she endlessly walks. It reminds me of Dad's sweeping away mannerism. The non-sequiturs in her speech, the aggression and non-cooperation. It all fits.

What has this realisation done to me? It has made me calmer. If this is what has happened, it is a monster neither she nor I can fight. It is something that has happened, that is irreversible, and it gives a physical explanation for her behaviour. No longer can I put it down to just being difficult.

Here's proof of its effect on me. Ironically, last night, the night after I got Alison's e-mail, there was a toilet disaster but throughout I remained calm, reassuring, encouraging. The net result of that is that, by and large, so did Bonnie. It is a stroke of some sort that has caused this, I am now utterly convinced, which means she really can't help any of it. That has helped me beyond measure.

Thinking about it as I write this, it must seem pretty weird that I am in effect saying I am glad that my darling Bonnie has had a mini-stroke. That shows how desperate things are. Pretty cruel disease, dementia, wouldn't you say? I have read that it can cause strokes, and it looks as if that is what it has done. Bon's son H says that the wiring in his mum's brain is fucked. What better non-medical description of a stroke can there be?

* * * *

I have started to tell certain people about my decision. Without exception, all are supportive, which is good. Many say they can't imagine what I am going through, which is true. I had an e-mail this morning from a medical colleague who has become a friend. She said it must be awful when someone you love is no longer in their own skin. That's pretty direct, but it sums it up perfectly. Boy, did I ever think that at breakfast just now. Bon wouldn't sit down and eat. Her tea was getting cold, her croissant slowly congealing, but each time Monika or I mentioned it, she said yes, yes, I know, I am doing it. In the end, we gave up. Who is this person inside my Bonnie's skin? Not my Bonnie, that's for sure.

* * * *

Mornings are worst. It seems every day begins with Bonnie in a bad mood. We came down this morning, the house bathed in sunlight. 'Beautiful, beautiful morning,' I said. 'I don't see why,' she said. 'Come on then, breakfast.' 'Breakfast, breakfast, breakfast, always breakfast.' And the look on her face a mixture of blankness and disinterest. Just not my Bonnie, nothing like my Bonnie, a different person.

Standing in her dressing gown as I write this, pacing the kitchen, gazing out to the garden uncomprehendingly. Now into the *séjour*, a glance at me tap-tapping, and out again. 'How are you darling?' and I curse myself for asking. 'Ooh, not too good,' in a slightly aggressive voice. I really should get her dressed, but I am not yet ready for the struggle.

* * * *

We have an ancient oak dining table in Tardan. I think I had better rephrase that. A local man who is a wonderful furniture maker custom-built us an oak dining table. When I asked him what size he would make it, he shrugged and said he would decide later. That's how they do things down here.

We came down a couple of months later to find it in place. No discussion with us of where we wanted it, how near to this wall or that wall, and when I looked at it I thought he had decided to sell us an antique table. It was battered, bruised, with woodworm trails all over it. We were both thrilled – far better an antique table than something new that didn't go with an old farmhouse. My only concern was that if the woodworm were active, they might leap out of the table into our ceiling beams.

When Francis came round, I asked him excitedly how old the table was. He looked a bit confused, then realised why I had asked, and said, 'Hah! It is new! As I promised you! I made it!' He patiently explained how he had tempered the solid oak, using a machine to score the wood-worm trails, and put the stress marks in by walking round bashing the table with a hammer.

How we adore our table! I can't count how many meals with family and friends we have had round it over the years, how much laughter has reverberated across it, how much wine and candle wax has spilled on it. We used to believe it possessed some spiritual quality. It was Bonnie who said one year, 'I think it has something to do with the width. It is not too wide, not too narrow. It brings people together.'

I have written countless words about Beethoven sitting at this table. I never expected to be writing about Bonnie in the way I am while sitting at it.

✳ ✳ ✳ ✳

Jean-Pierre and Claudette came round last night. Bonnie greeted them aggressively. 'I know who they are, I know what to do,' she said, failing to give them the customary French *bisou*. While we sat with an aperitif, she just walked and walked. Claudette couldn't believe how much she had deteriorated since the last time we were here, just over a month ago.

'*Pauvre John*,' said Jean-Pierre as they left. That hit me. In bed I allowed myself a little bit of self-pity. Fortunately, sleep came quickly.

✳ ✳ ✳ ✳

Bonnie will not sit through a meal now. She gets up and walks around after a few mouthfuls. If Monika or I say something, she gets angry and says of course she will eat her meal, but she just keeps walking.

Gave her the iPod and Abba this afternoon. Boy, she loves Abba. As soon as she hears those harmonies and infectious beat, she is happy. She sings along. Same with Frank Sinatra, Nat King Cole and Barbra Streisand. They have always been favourites, and they still are. We share that. We also used to share Beethoven, obviously, but she doesn't ask for him any more. Fair enough, I don't push it. Sometimes I plug the iPod into the speakers so the sound reverberates round the house. Actually, I'm getting to quite like Abba.

So I put the Swedish phenomenon on the iPod for her and she walked round the whole afternoon, listening. Early evening, it had vanished. I looked everywhere. Went into the laundry room and the washing machine had leaked. My stomach sank. I *hate* it when appliances break down. It's always such a nightmare getting the service engineer, even in London, and I've never had to do it down here in France.

But then I realised the machine hadn't leaked and I was almost relieved. I stayed calm, got Bon into the shower while Monika mopped up. She emerged from the laundry room clutching the iPod. Bon had put it in a plastic basin of dirty clothes.

More weight to the small stroke theory. I kept calm. It has gone way beyond something she can control.

We went to the covered market in Aire-sur-l'Adour today. God, how Bon used to run around that market, jostling with the locals, selecting the best this and the best that – white nectarines that were like eating sugar, small flat peaches that came from heaven, avocadoes perfectly ready, artichokes (which I always cooked, very complicated, place in pan, fill with water, add salt, bring to the boil, allow to simmer for one hour, serve *without anything, no oil and vinegar, no Italian dressing, nothing*), ewe's cheese from the Pyrenees, local blue cheese (which the stall lady told us to add to green salad), duck, duck and duck. Now she walked uncomprehendingly, getting tetchy when I guided her in the right direction. We walked back along the main street to the car, passing the estate agent and its window in which we saw that faded Polaroid 20 years ago almost to the day. No point in saying anything.

I am being inundated with requests to speak at dementia conferences in the autumn. Seven in six weeks. Mr Dementia, Mr Carer, that's me. Not a role I ever foresaw for myself. I should say yes to them all – it'll raise awareness (that is now such a universal cliché – *'raise bloody awareness'*), will be of help to other carers, and keep me busy in the weeks following losing Bon to Sundial. I also know it'll help my charity, *for dementia*.

So I'll probably say yes. But do you know what I really *really* want to do? Go and live in a garret in Paris, grow a beard, play jazz trombone badly, and die of absinthe poisoning.

I have started listening to Willie Nelson and Johnny Cash. There is no hope for me.

I am dreaming of Bonnie more and more often, and it is my Bonnie of the glory days. I don't have to explain what the dreams are about. It is obvious. So vivid, so totally vivid. It used to be such a wonderful feeling waking up that way. Reach out, feel arms encircle me, a sigh of comprehension. Now I keep very still, knowing that the slightest movement will wake her up, and it is off to attend to toilet duties. This Bonnie is no longer my Bonnie. How can I cope with that? I suppose it might make it easier to handle the dreaded event of September 15th. Might.

I'm not sleeping well down here in France. I wake up at 3.30 or 4 in the morning, and that's it for a couple of hours. Why? No doubt too much wine at dinner, but exacerbated certainly by worries about the future. And those worries are never more acute than in the dead dark stillness of the night.

What if Bonnie doesn't settle at Sundial? What do I do then? Tough it out, or bring her home? What about me? Friends and family all urge me to fill my life, look after myself, plan a future. But how will I be when Bonnie has actually moved out of my life? I will go to visit her like a patient in a hospital. What will I think in the dead of night then? What should I do about this old house of so many memories? Should I sell it? I know the boys want it for their kids, but they are not ready yet. I can't come on my own, not for long periods anyway, so it will remain closed up. Not good. But we are in a recession, nobody is buying anything, let alone huge old farmhouses in deepest France. What about the flat? Should I move out of it, our home for all our married life (and more)? Will I need the memories to wallow in, or should I start again? I am 65. Yesterday it was announced a top Hollywood director and screenwriter (*Ferris Bueller's Day Off*, the *Home Alone* series) died suddenly of a heart attack at 59.

All these questions. John, the Great Planner, everything neatly worked out. Not any more. My life at the moment, August 2009, is a series of question marks.

I've blown my top over the dementia conferences. An eighth, can you believe that? All in the first few weeks after Bon goes into Sundial. It's ridiculous. The dementia industry are world champion conference holders. Well, I have said no, and I'll probably say no to a load I have already said yes to. It all depends on how Bon settles in to Sundial. What if it's a disaster? What if I have to bring her home again? Then it's no to everything. Simple as that. They can have their conferences without me.

*   *   *   *

The usual shower ritual nightmare this morning. 'I don't want a shower, I'm not having a shower, I'm not taking my dressing gown off.' This time I got angry, but in a controlled way. 'Right, enough of this nonsense.' I took her dressing gown off her, she protested for a moment, then did exactly as I said. Maybe the path of least resistance is not always the answer.

I had the bathroom here redone a year ago, and the shower is a nice spacious walk-in one. Room for two. Just think – *just think!* – what we might have got up to in the old days.

The shower wall is made of glass tiles. The tiler joked with me how nice it would be to watch a beautiful woman having a shower through the glass wall. I watched Bonnie this morning, muttering to herself, complaining when I told her to use soap. In our bedsit in Washington, the shower was a glass cubicle. Bonnie posed for me in it, showering, soaping, pressing herself against the glass. I took photographs. They are hidden somewhere at the back of one of the cupboards in the flat.

Sometimes I envy her loss of memory.

*   *   *   *

I am an inveterate day counter. It goes back to my awful boarding school days. In term time I used to count the days gleefully to going home on holiday, on holiday I used to count the days sadly before going back to school. Now I am counting the days to 27th August – 13 – when we drive away from here, and beyond it to the fateful date of 15th September. Life doesn't change much, does it?

We were sitting on the terrace this afternoon when our immediate neighbour Annie came round. We kissed on both cheeks, but Bonnie was reluctant, saying rather aggressively, 'They're always kissing here. It's stupid.' Annie was not offended. She wanted to ask my permission to clear away an old apple tree of ours, which had fallen across her back hedge. I hadn't even noticed, other things on my mind. She brought some small peaches she had picked for us. Bon tucked in. When I suggested she thanked Annie, she got angry.

Annie and I chatted. She lost her husband a few years ago, and towards the end he had had dementia. He was in his early eighties, but she said she understood. Of course she doesn't really, but I appreciated her sympathy. I asked her, in French, if she could tell that Bonnie had deteriorated. *'Ah oui,'* she said with startling directness, *'c'est fini.'*

Claudette came round a few hours later. *'Qu'est-ce qu'elle a changé,'* she kept saying, *'qu'est-ce qu'elle a changé.'*

This is no longer my Bonnie. Not the way my Bonnie talks, walks, laughs, behaves, eats, anything, everything. I am living with a different person inside my Bonnie's body, and that is the person who will be going into Sundial in just over a month from now.

Bonnie used to be like an informal agony aunt. Friends, colleagues, anyone who knew her would gravitate to her to spill out their problems. I remember back in the Henley days, sometime in the mid or late 1970s (long before 'The Kiss'), she and her husband invited my wife and me up to their house for New Year's Eve.

As you can imagine, I was counting the days, hours, then minutes until it was time to go up the slope. There were a few other couples there as well, whom I didn't know. The champagne was soon flowing, I began to feel that warmth in my veins, and my eyes swivelled dangerously towards the beautiful American blonde with the Grace Kelly looks. Suddenly I saw one of the other husbands, a tall bloke with a ridiculous Abe Lincoln beard, raise an eyebrow to Bonnie, and the two of them walked down the corridor to the kitchen.

Soon they were engaged in intense conversation. I could just see the silhouettes of their faces, their hands every now and then gesticulating. It was clear he was doing most of the talking. I can't remember much more about the evening, except that I practically didn't see either of them again. They must have come back into the living room, and joined us all for the buffet dinner, I can't remember. My abiding memory is that they spent the entire evening in the kitchen in intense conversation, and I didn't exchange two words with my fantasy female. It was obvious to me that the man was in love with her, he was declaring that love, and he was trying to persuade her to reciprocate, to have an affair with him. It made for the most depressing start to a new year that I could imagine.

Soon after the miracle happened and Bonnie and I were at last together, I asked her about that evening. 'That bearded wonder, was he trying to have an affair with you?' She didn't understand at first, then the penny dropped and she laughed out loud. 'No,' she said, 'it was nothing like that. He was telling me that his marriage was in a bit of trouble, he just felt he and his wife were falling out of love, and he was pouring his heart out to me.'

'Yeah,' I said cynically, 'trying to have an affair with you.' 'No, honestly,' she said, 'it really wasn't like that.' She must have been right and she must have given the man good advice, because I heard from the couple after I went public about Bonnie's illness. They were still married and were now grandparents.

* * * *

I have heard from my pen friend Jim up in Bolton. Jan is very aggressive, lashes out at him, and from what he describes she has far more difficult toilet issues than Bon. She attends a day centre three days a week to give Jim some respite, but they have now told Jim she can't attend on Wednesdays, when they are busiest, because she has become too aggressive.

There are people in my situation, some better off than me, some a lot worse off. Bon is not physically aggressive (even if sneezing is no longer quite the most aggressive thing she ever does), just difficult and uncooperative.

Someone I respect said to me in an e-mail that she thinks I have thought through everything incredibly lovingly and thoroughly, and taken myself to the brink of what a partner can cope with.

Is she right? If she is, it's very encouraging to read that. But Jim has taken things further, hasn't he? If he can, why can't I?

What a wonderful moment just now! I crouched on the floor here in the *séjour* to plug the laptop cable into the wall. I had to reach behind some furniture, and it wasn't easy. I heard Bon laugh from the other end of the room as she saw my predicament. I pretended to be stuck. 'Help,' I cried. 'I'm stuck, I can't get up.'

'I'm coming, I'm coming,' she said, laughing out loud as she hurried across the room. 'Quick, quick!' I said. 'Help, help!' 'Here I am, here I am!' She bent down, put her hands on my side, and pulled gently upwards. I stood effortlessly. 'Thank you so much,' I said. 'If you hadn't helped me, I'd still be down there tonight.' She laughed, I put my arms round her and gave her a big hug, and she reciprocated! Golden moment.

Less than a week from now, I go back to London for two days to present a Prom on BBC Television. Beethoven's *Fidelio*. I accepted it earlier this year with glee. I will talk about Beethoven to anyone, anywhere, at any time. But now I am dreading it. Why? Because it is the ultimate love story. Woman is prepared to lay down her life to save her husband's. There is a moment after the climax when they clasp each other, reunited, safe, which always makes me cry. 'Oh Leonore,' Florestan asks, 'what have you done for me?' 'Nothing, nothing at all, my Florestan,' she replies, and the strings soar for the opening of a glorious hymn to love, *O namenlose Freude*, [Oh joy beyond words]. This, composed by a man who never found lasting love. How am I going to talk about this wonderful work of art live on television without the tears coming?

I have just spent the afternoon listening to *Fidelio* on the terrace. When it got to that moment after Leonore saves her husband's life, and says she has done nothing, I lost it, completely lost it. Great tears rolling down my cheeks. How am I going to cope at the Prom? All right, I'll be off camera at that point, but surrounded by BBC producers and VIPs, and I'll sit there blubbing.

In the final chorus, Florestan sings of how any man who has found such a wife should rejoice for ever. He calls her *Retterin* [saviour]. How many times has Bonnie saved me from myself, from my impetuosity, my impatience? And how am I paying her back? By putting her into a home. A month from today. I am about to embark on the worst month of my life.

Now I watch her walking up and down the kitchen, in her dressing gown, hat and scarf, listening to Abba on the iPod, her right hand clutching the gown behind her. At least she is walking upright. Ah my Bonnie, my *Retterin*, why did you have to leave me?

I stroked her on the back just now, then moved my hand down and stroked her bottom. 'Right, that is enough, John,' she said. Now that really *IS NOT* my Bonnie.

Monika said this morning, 'You are being killed from inside by the memories.' Is there a better way of putting it? I don't think so.

I flew to London for just two days to do the *Fidelio* prom for the BBC. I blubbed my way through most of it, fortunately off camera. I phoned Monika back in Tardan on the first day, and she said Bonnie had been in a difficult mood and there had been an incontinence attack. Fortunately it was on the tiled kitchen floor, so easy to deal with. The second day – yesterday – Bonnie had been much more amenable. Both nights went without problem.

But the most significant factor is that Bonnie did not mention me once while I was away. Monika even sat in my chair (mine for the past 20 years) at the kitchen table, and still Bon did not mention me. She didn't ask where I had gone, why I wasn't there, or anything.

We can get BBC Television down here in France. Monika told me she put the Prom on last night. Bon sat watching it with her. When my mug popped up, Monika asked Bon if she recognised who that was. Bon said no, but she was sure he was very well known.

Half of me is heartbroken, but the other half is not. Further sign – maybe – that she will settle in Sundial well. Maybe. Perhaps.

I have had a repeat of what happened to me in Krakow. Two nights after the stress of the Prom, I lay awake most of the night with searing stomach pains. This morning it was worse. I sat at the kitchen table stretched back in agony. Monika pleaded with me to call an ambulance. I put it off, put it off, put it off. But the pain worsened. Then, around 10.30, as if by magic, a small expulsion of air, nothing dramatic, and minutes later the pain dissipated as if by magic. One moment about to call an ambulance, the next no pain at all.

But it's a worry. Why did it happen? I had no alcohol at all last night, and Monika cooked a lovely chicken dinner – nothing spicy or hot. Does it mean the Polish doctor was right, and it wasn't the pills that caused it in Krakow? I had better do the round of the quacks again. Stress is the only thing I can think of. The Prom was incredibly stressful, but it was good stress. Live television, it's what I thrive on. But is my body telling me, come on, old man, time to stop putting yourself through all this? If it is, God help me when it comes to the dementia conferences in October/November. Now that really will be stressful.

I suppose it didn't help that when I was looking for the television remote last night, I finally found it hidden in one of Bon's slippers. She saw me find it. 'There,' she said triumphantly, 'I knew you'd be pleased. I was keeping it safe.'

Bonnie, by the way, did not react in any way to seeing me doubled-up in pain. She did not comprehend, and so just continued her walking.

The timing couldn't have been worse. Roughly 15 years ago, we had a long Easter weekend booked in Prague. Beethoven research. Thursday, the day before we flew, I was due to present the lunchtime news on ITN. Around 11 o'clock, I began to feel nauseous. A dull stomach ache that was slowly worsening. I'd eaten and drunk nothing out of the normal either the previous night or at breakfast, yet I felt increasingly ill. The last time I felt like this was at school after I drank an entire carton of condensed milk.

A soothing cup of herbal tea made things worse. I looked at the computer screen, across to the studio, behind to the door leading to the toilets. I really thought I was about to throw up. I felt absolutely dreadful, yet I had a live news programme to present in a little over an hour, and a flight to Prague early the next morning.

I had never done it before, not once in my entire career, but I knew I couldn't go on. Unsteadily I crossed the newsroom to the admin desk. Pauline looked up at me and gasped. 'Are you all right? You're white as a sheet.' 'I don't know why, but I feel dreadfully sick.' 'Go home,' she said. 'I'll call a car for you. Go home now.'

I phoned Bon before I left. 'I'll leave work early. Don't worry. I'll be home soon.'

I got home and went straight to bed, my stomach feeling as if it were full of unset cement.

Today, as I sit here writing about it, I can *see* Bonnie walk into the bedroom, slipping off her brown leather coat with the slightly gathered shoulders (she hadn't wanted to buy it, but I knew it suited her, and she wore it for 10 years until it practically fell off her), cross to the bed and sit gently alongside me. She felt my slightly damp forehead and stroked my hair. Out of the room, and back in a minute or so with a cool flannel. She wiped the cold beads away and stroked my cheeks.

'I'm here now. I'll look after you, my darling,' she said. And I knew everything would be fine.

* * * *

We drive away from Tardan in two days, and I am in hunkered-down, brace-myself mode. I e-mailed a friend and told him about Bonnie not recognising me on television. He wrote back to say that if ever I needed it, that is the conclusive proof that she is ready for full-time care. 'It proves you have taken things as far as you possibly can,' he wrote. 'In fact, a lot further than many men in your position would have done.'

That made me feel … well, I wouldn't say good, but maybe a little better. Our neighbours Raymonde and Michou invited us round for drinks last night. They knew it was the last time they would spend with Bonnie, and after 20 years they wanted to see her. Bon sat the whole time saying nothing, eating all the nibbles they had put out. They told me in French how sad the whole thing was, and how they totally understood my decision.

Their daughter is getting married at the end of September. We are, of course, invited. Bonnie will be in Sundial, and I told them weeks ago that obviously we wouldn't be able to come. Then I thought about it, and why the hell shouldn't I come? A three-day break down here, in the house alone without Bon for the first time, but a wedding to go to, lots of drinking, eating and dancing. Everybody will know how I feel inside and will do their best to give me a good time.

I ran it past Raymonde and Michou and they threw their arms up in pleasure. So I am coming down for the wedding – *tout seul*. Bon will have been in Sundial for just 10 days. If it turns out to be a complete disaster and I have to take her out again, then obviously I won't come down. But she seems so amenable and calm, if that happened it would surprise me. It is something for me to look forward to, beyond the dreadful date of 15th September.

The weather has turned grey and gloomy. It is due to stay this way till we go on Thursday. Then the forecast is for the return of warm sunny weather. Seems appropriate.

* * * *

The last afternoon on the terrace, I listened to *Tannhäuser*. (Great Teutonic hero chooses eternal love over earthly pleasures. Or stupid German gives up guaranteed sex with any woman he wants in pursuit of unattainable goddess. Take your pick. Either way, he dies.) Bon just walked in and out of the house.

We went round to say goodbye to Jean-Pierre and Claudette. They were aware it was probably the last time they would see Bon. They kept strong faces, but at the last moment I saw their eyes moisten.

I keep telling myself this is not the Bonnie I shared this house with for all those years; she has already left. Now I am leaving with a different person who happens to exist inside Bonnie's body.

The last dinner, last glass of wine, last night in the house together. Being a man, I got drunk. Bit stupid, really.

Goodbye to the house, the trees we planted. Bon got quietly into the car, oblivious to it all. I was fine, until I closed the gate behind me. Quick cry, then back into the car. It helps that I am coming back in a month for the wedding.

So that's a big hurdle crossed. I have left Tardan with Bonnie for the last time. Now for 15th September. Not so much a hurdle, more a high jump.

Chapter 14

My head's in a mess. August bank holiday weekend. Two weeks and two days to Sundial. We sat watching TV last night, the *Catherine Tate Show*. Bon laughed like a drain. She got every joke. (Not that they're exactly subtle.) Am I making a massive mistake, one that is going to ruin my lovely Bonnie's life? *Why are we here? Why are you leaving me? Where are we? What is going on?* That is my night and day nightmare.

I have had to order name tapes for Bonnie's clothes. Monika said she would sew them in. Last time I saw that happen was when my Mum sewed name tapes into my clothes for boarding school.

* * * *

Fantasy in B minor

'Look, it's September, there's glorious sunshine, let's go to a Greek island for a week.'

'Ah, wonderful idea! You book the flights and the hotel, I'll do all the packing. And I know just what you want me to wear — and not wear.'

'We can swim nude together, sunbathe on empty beaches. We'll eat grilled sardines for lunch and drink Retsina.'

'It'll be a second honeymoon. I can't wait.'

* * * *

Gruelling day. Began with a visit to our GP. She told me putting Bonnie into a home would give me closure of a sort, and I must use it to rebuild my life and move on. But it won't be easy, she said. I will be overwhelmed with emotion. 'If you want to cry, cry,' she said, 'don't hold it in.' Then she said something that took me aback. 'Some people will feel that you are doing the wrong thing, that you shouldn't be putting Bonnie into a home. Whatever they say to your face, that is what they will be feeling. You must take no notice, not even think of it. You are doing the right thing, both for her and you.'

Is that right? Will some people think that? Just the thought of it drags me down. It'll make me think twice when someone says to me, 'Oh yes, you are doing absolutely the right thing.' Are they actually thinking '*selfish bastard*'? They'd better keep it to themselves in that case.

Then to John Lewis in Oxford Street to furnish Bonnie's room. I took Monika, because I thought she might have an idea or two. Just as well I did. In the mid-1980s, Bon and I used to come to this store practically every weekend to furnish our flat. Now here I was, furnishing her single room in a home. I was weighed down by memories and just wanted to get out of the store. So I went into hyper-efficient, quick-decision, alpha-male mode, and chose the wrong bed, the wrong chest of drawers, the wrong chairs, the wrong bedside lamp. Monika quietly over-ruled every decision I made, and we ended up with the right stuff.

At one point I looked across the floor at some bookshelves, and my damned memory sent me back 25 years, standing in almost the same spot and gazing in the same direction. I saw Mum and Dad over by the shelving, looking at a bookcase. Their backs were to us. I nudged Bon, she looked over and smiled. 'Don't disturb them,' she said. I nodded. Dad was in his late seventies, Mum seventy-one or two. We watched them for a few minutes, then they moved off. I turned to Bonnie. 'That'll be us one day,' I said.

I held up until the final item, a picture for the wall opposite her bed. Many years ago Bonnie bought me an oil painting of poppies for my birthday, and it has hung on the wall opposite our bed in the flat ever since. We love the fact that it is like a window set into the wall, giving us a beautiful rural view of bright red poppies, a stream meandering down the side of the frame. It is painted as if the artist is lying among the poppies.

In the picture section there was a picture of poppies in a field. Not the same as ours, but poppies in a field nonetheless. 'That's the one,' I said, and the tears came.

* * * *

We have some good friends, Judith and Maurice, who live just along the corridor from us in our block of flats. Judith rang and asked if we could all go out to dinner. I decided to go round and bring them up to date. They knew I had been thinking of full-time care for Bonnie, but didn't know it was now less than two weeks away.

Judith, who was a nurse, said it was absolutely the right decision. She had known a man in a similar position to me, who had kept his wife at home for years. She finally died when he was 75. His health was broken by then, Judith said, he had nothing else to live for, no outside interests, no friends, nothing, so followed her soon after. 'You mustn't let that happen to you,' she said.

Maurice then said something that really shocked me. 'The first time we noticed there was anything wrong was when we all went to the Royal Academy of Music for a concert. Must have been at least five years ago, 2003 or 2004. Do you remember? You were working, and you said you would join us a bit late. So Bonnie took us, led us into the hall and we sat down. Only problem was there was no one else there, no music stands, nothing. She said it was definitely the right place. We sat for 10 or 15 minutes before I said I would just go and have a look around, and of course we were in the wrong hall. But at the time, we put it down to a simple mistake.'

That's it exactly. Things start to happen, and you put them down to simple error, a misunderstanding, a moment of forgetfulness, you even make jokes about losing your marbles. But in reality it is the early stages of a dreadful, dreadful journey.

✳ ✳ ✳ ✳

My niece Katherine is getting married tomorrow. Wedding in the White Tower of the Tower of London. Huge family get-together. I have been worried about it for weeks. The ceremony is at 4pm, with reception to follow. Since I made the decision on Sundial, I have seen it as Bonnie's last major family outing – a chance for her to see them and them to see her 10 days before she goes in.

But as things have deteriorated with Bon, I've become increasingly anxious. In discussion with David, I decided that we would, of course, come to the service, but that Monika would bring Bon home afterwards. I would stay on for the reception, but if things proved difficult I would come home as well, then leave after a suitable interval and return for the reception.

Got up this morning. Accident on the bathroom floor. Not horrendous, more a nuisance than anything. Bon blissfully unaware. But it meant the day began with me in deep depression. At breakfast, I said to Monika (Bonnie was walking up and down the corridor) that I was worried about the wedding. What if there was an accident?

Monika said, 'John, it is better that she does not go. I will stay with her here in the flat. You go. You will be more relaxed.' I looked at her stunned. It simply had not occurred to me. 'Ridiculous. Don't be silly,' I said, a little too sharply. 'She must come. It's the last time …'

My head sank between my shoulders. Of course, it was the answer. Obvious. 'Yes,' I said, 'you're right.'

I am relating this only because the moment I made the decision, it was as if a ton weight had come off my shoulders. I felt free. I smiled. If

Bonnie were not at the wedding, there would be no problems. It was not as if the family would mind – they all understood exactly what was going on. It also freed me from potential emotional embarrassment, watching Bonnie pretty lost among family she had known for almost 30 years. I might still find it a bit hard being there without her, but that would be easier to handle than having to keep a constant watch out for problems.

So, decision made. I won't say anything, I'll just change, Monika will distract Bonnie, and I will go. Breaks my heart, but that's not exactly a new feeling, is it?

* * * *

I went to the wedding on my own. Lots of sympathy, concern, family all around. 'Don't feel guilty,' I kept being told. It doesn't really help, because I knew I had to come back to the flat and climb into bed next to Bonnie, who had no idea of where I had been.

* * * *

Wait! Stop! Hold the front page! Hold everything! Yes, ladies and gentlemen, sound the trumpets, beat the drum, the front page of today's *Daily Mail* proudly declares: ALZHEIMER'S: A MASSIVE LEAP.

Yes, 'British scientists have made the biggest breakthrough for more than 15 years in the fight against Alzheimer's … Their landmark research *could* revolutionise … It *could* cut the rate of new cases … The research has also raised the *possibility* that Alzheimer's … This means anti-inflammatory medicines *could* help … It is *possible* the changes in these genes … It *could* take years to find the right chemicals for a drug … Experts do *not yet* have enough information for a genetic test, but one is *likely* to be developed … Most importantly the research *could* also lead to new drug treatments.' [My italics.]

Or not. It is to do with identifying rogue genes responsible for one in five cases of the disease. Or, more accurately, one in five of 6,000 Alzheimer's sufferers among 16,000 people who took part in the study.

So take my advice, all ye who care, or suffer, or fear that one day you might care or suffer. Don't hold your breath.

* * * *

Wednesday 9th September, six days before Bonnie goes into Sundial. John Lewis have just telephoned me to say all the furniture has been delivered. 'We've unpacked everything and put it in the room,' the helpful deliveryman told me. 'You may want to move it about a bit, but it's all there.' I thanked him profusely for putting my mind at rest.

Bonnie was sitting next to me when I took the call on my mobile. As I rang off, I said, 'Excellent news.' 'Oh good,' she said.

It got to me a bit. She didn't know that her new (single) bed, chest of drawers and easy chairs had been delivered to the room she will be moving into next week. She was just pleased that I was pleased. I had to walk down the corridor of the flat a bit to stifle a small choke, but I had to be quick about it because I knew she wouldn't be far behind me.

We watched some anarchic comedy on TV in the evening, then time to get ready for bed. She was happy and laughing, so was I.

Into the bathroom, teeth first, then the toilet. She sat, waited, waited, waited, fumbling with her clothes, up down up down up down. Finally success. I handed her paper. She used it, but clothes up down up down up down, soiled paper in hand. I began to get tense, but forced myself to stay calm. *Throw the paper away, throw it away.* I snatched it and threw it away. I stopped her fumbling with her clothes, and pulled up undies and slacks. *Right, bedroom,* and I left the bathroom. But she took clothes down again and sat on the toilet. I pulled her off it, pulled her clothes back up, and almost frog-marched her to the bedroom. Worst thing I could have done. She was now in total confusion, take clothes off, put them back on, take them off, put them back on. I finally tore her slacks down and got her, none too gently, into bed.

In the space of 15 minutes, I had gone from being happy and laughy to being at the end of my tether. I wanted to self-harm. I wanted to bang my head against the doorframe until I knocked myself out. Instead I went out into the corridor and let out a strangulated scream. It hurt my throat so much I can barely speak.

I must remember this in five days' time when I am alone, with no one to put to bed but myself.

* * * *

Zoe and Louise from Sundial came to the flat today to meet Bonnie. They wanted to see her *in situ*, to get an idea of how she lived and to try to discover something of her personality. In fact, as with all professionals, they spent relatively little time talking to her, but were able to make a remarkably detailed assessment.

I then took them into the dining room, while Monika distracted Bonnie, and we talked for the best part of three hours. They said so many wise things and I learned so much.

Remember, they said, that Bonnie will undergo a change in status when she comes to Sundial. I looked confused. Here, in the flat, they said, she is the most dependent person. She looks to me for everything, takes her cues from me, eats food prepared by Monika, takes her mood from me. In Sundial she will be better than most other residents, so she will sense her status is raised. She will realise this, they said, and it should make her feel better about herself, and help her adapt to her new environment and form friendships.

Furthermore, whatever she does will be right. I looked confused again (it comes naturally). They explained, patiently, that here in the flat obviously she can make mistakes, from the extreme case of incontinence, to not using her knife when she eats. In Sundial she will never do anything wrong. We are the ones who will have to learn from her. She is correct in everything she does: we have to adapt. Again, that will help her self-esteem.

I have to admit, all this was making me feel a hell of a lot better. These were professional care workers, with years of experience of looking after people with dementia. Every case of dementia is different, but already they were making it clear to me that looking after Bonnie was going to be no problem for them. 'Just think,' said Louise, 'you will never have to worry again.'

I asked them about my behaviour, how I should behave at Sundial, what sort of things I should say, how to come and go, and so on. They said one of their care staff had come up with a marvellous description of how a carer, a loved one, should behave. 'Parachute in, evaporate out.'

I laughed in pleasant shock at the sheer aptness of that. Arrive unannounced, and leave in the same way. The care staff would be all around. I should treat them like old friends from Day One, just give them the nod when I was about to leave, and they would take care of everything.

Remember too, Zoe said, the care staff work seven-hour shifts, no longer, and they don't take their work home with them. You have been living with this for 24 hours a day for many years, with things getting progressively worse. Plus Bonnie is the woman you love and the woman you married. The care staff have none of those burdens, which means they are in a far better position to care for Bonnie. As each day goes by, they will get to know Bonnie better and better, and after a month, one of them – whoever Bon has taken a particular shine to, and vice versa – will be appointed her designated care manager.

Naïve I certainly am. I thought putting someone into a home was a simple case of putting someone into a home. It is much, much more professional than that.

They stressed that I should look after myself, build a new life. I told them about the constant friend perched on my shoulder, the guilt demon. They said no, I must not feel guilt. I then remembered something Bonnie had said to me many years ago, and I repeated it. 'If anything happened to me,' she said, 'you'd have the time of your life and you'd marry again, and quite right too.' In unison, Zoe and Louise said, 'She has given you consent.'

I swallowed hard. Really? When Bonnie said that, was that what she meant? I doubted it. 'Would she want you to be happy or sad?' asked Zoe. 'If it was the other way round, would you want her to be happy or sad?' asked Louise. I gave in to their argument gracefully.

'One final thing,' Louise said, 'Sundial is a happy place. We don't walk around with long faces, nor do the residents. People with dementia are, on the whole, very contented people.' I knew that was true of Bonnie. 'And we have a lot of laughs,' she said.

Then the stories came tumbling out. 'Never eat chocolate drops in a dementia unit. Golden rule, after one of the residents rolled her poo into perfect little balls, put them in a chocolate box, and offered them to a carer … What about the dear old chap, so spick and span, always wears a tie, and takes out his toothbrush to comb his hair? … Or the lovely old dear whose favourite colour is pink, she wears a pink suit, pink blouse, and one day her daughters smuggled in some pink nail varnish (against the rules, imagine if a resident drank it) and hid it, intending to paint their mother's nails next time they came in, but she found it, and painted her teeth a perfect pink to go with her suit … And the poor care worker who came to me at the end of the day and said I have had a shit day – turned out Mrs So-and-So, owner of a beautiful long-necked vase, had put her poo in small pieces down it, for some reason water wouldn't dislodge it, and only this carer had small enough hands to fish it all out.'

Zoe, Louise and I, talking about dementia, the cruellest disease in the world, my Bonnie about to go into Sundial where they would look after her, all creased up laughing at poo jokes.

I suppose it's a week of 'lasts'. I took Bonnie to our local Chinese this evening (Friday). We have been going there for more than 10 years, we know them, they know us. I gave Bon a birthday party a few years ago in the private room, and there was a huge Suchet family party in the same room early in 2008. We have had many laughs in the place.

Tonight Bonnie was uncooperative, aggressive, rude, criticised everything I said, disagreed with my choice of dishes (for the last four or five years, she has always willingly let me order for her). My blasted memory again. I looked across at her, that sullen face, and saw in my mind's eye the laughing angel who almost fell off the chair with hilarity when I told her colleague and wife that we looked across a crowded room and said 'Ugh' to each other because we were not very good with words. By the time we left the Chinese, I didn't know whether to scream out loud or burst into tears.

Back in the flat, got her ready for bed, would she spend a penny? Would she hell. Three times she sat down and got up again. At the end of my tether, I lay down across the bathroom doorway and told her she was going nowhere until she spent a penny. She tried twice more, without success. I actually fell asleep. Finally Monika came to the rescue and put her to bed. I went and sat in an armchair and blubbed like a baby. I knew I would be waking up to a massive clean-up.

It's not that this woman inhabiting my Bonnie's body is no longer my Bonnie, it's that this woman *is no longer my Bonnie.* Do you know how utterly awful that is? Can you begin to imagine?

It's morning now, and guess what? All was fine. Up as normal six-ish, did everything – no paper, no washing, but what the hell. So all my histrionics and melodramatics were a waste of time. I hurt Bonnie and I hurt myself for no reason.

Dementia does not teach you about the person with dementia, it teaches you about yourself. Believe me, you do not like all you find. I obviously have a cruel, vicious side to my character that is deep down and dormant, that I didn't know I had. Or do I? Is it rather something that only comes into existence under certain extreme circumstances, and is not actually part of my character?

That's one for the physichrists (as Dad used to call them). Too deep for my simple mind.

* * * *

Our last walk in Regent's Park. I didn't take us across the lake and up the slope, where we went on that first walk together nearly 27 years ago. Not for any sentimental reason, but because the air was chilly and Bonnie would get cold if we went too far. So we walked along the side of the lake, not saying much. There's no conversation any more. I made my usual jokes about the birds beating each other up and the gentle scent of goose poo in the air. Then I took Bon for her morning hot chocolate, again for the last time.

Sunday night. Late. My brother Pete called earlier to say he was thinking of me ahead of Tuesday. David and his wife Sheila came round this afternoon. He's got all kinds of plans for my future. Damian rang me and said he, Kieran and H were going to take me out to dinner on Tuesday. I resisted. They said there was no way I was going to be alone. Can't beat family, it's like a warm protective wall around you.

* * * *

Everything is a 'last' now. Dinner, bed, sleep, up tomorrow, breakfast. I went out to Sundial today, Monday, and got her room ready. Bed made, poppy picture up, TV tuned, cupboard filled with her clothes. Damp eyes throughout. But as I left, I saw her name on a small plaque by the door: Mrs Bonnie Suchet. That did it. Tears.

Louise was on hand to hug me and cheer me up. 'Are you in the habit of bringing Bonnie flowers?' she asked with a glint in her eye. I was a bit thrown. 'Well, I haven't for a while,' I said slightly guiltily. 'Why? Is there a policy? Can I bring flowers?' 'Only if they're edible,' she said. We both creased up with laughter. 'I mean it,' she said. 'Not that Bonnie will try to eat them, but you'll be surprised how many residents do.' And we creased up again.

Louise said I would take it far more badly tomorrow than Bonnie. I just hope that is the case.

Tears are constantly pricking behind my eyes. My skin feels sore, as if the nerves underneath have had their ends shaved off. I must hold it together when I leave the flat with her tomorrow morning. She will be leaving it for the last time, this flat that has witnessed virtually our entire 26 years together.

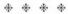

Can you believe this? Can you honestly believe it? This morning, this crucial morning that will change my life and my Bonnie's life forever, in the hour or so before I woke up I had an erotic dream about another woman. I honestly did. A rather beautiful woman I know, so a real woman, not just a fantasy figure. We were together in a hotel room, we both knew what was about to happen, we moved slowly, I breathed in the scent on her neck, raised my hand to turn her face towards me, and Bonnie stirred in the bed for her first early trip to the toilet. It was 6.30.

Guilt descended on me like a ton of bricks, then I smiled. It wasn't Bonnie in the dream, but the hotel room, the slow-motion movement ... It was the Harley in New York, 1982. How memory can mess you up!

At breakfast the weather forecaster on the telly said the day in the south-east would be 'grey, damp and drizzly'. Pretty appropriate, I thought. I repeated what she had said. 'Grey, damp and drizzly,' I said. 'Yes,' said Bonnie, 'and if you don't watch out I might do that to you some day.' I smiled. I peeled an expertly (machine) boiled egg for her, and at breakfast could not help thinking we had survived the night with no accidents. I would not have to deal with any more accidents again.

Then I caught sight of the little 'Bonnie's Kitchen' sign hanging from the cooker hood, which I had bought for her and hung there after we had the kitchen redone in 1988. As I have said before, it is the little things that crack you up.

The case was packed, she let me put her into her warm coat, hat and scarf, never once asking why. I told her we were going away for a short break. 'Good,' she said.

At 11 o'clock we left the flat. Tears brimmed in my eyes. At the last moment, Monika shoved a small packet of tissues into my hand. We walked the oh-so-familiar street to Marylebone station. There I bought her a single ticket. Oh yes, it's those little things that crack you up.

Into a taxi at the other end, and to Sundial. Louise was there waiting for us and whisked us straight to the second floor. I kept saying how beautiful the place was. Bonnie caught sight of the first very elderly dementia sufferer, and then another. She shot me a look as if to say, 'Blimey, they're a bit past it.' 'Thank God for us young 'uns,' I said. She laughed.

A crucial moment approached. How would she react to her room, her single room with single bed? We walked in and I said, 'Isn't this lovely?' 'Yes,' she said. 'Look at the amazing view,' I said. 'Yes, it's lovely,' she replied.

I unpacked, she used the toilet successfully, and seemed really happy. Louise took us into the dining room for lunch. Very elderly people all around. Bon looked a bit bemused, but remained in good spirits. She ate well, and made no adverse comments.

After lunch we sat in two easy chairs in the large communal area and Louise brought us coffee. Bon was becoming a little restless. 'So many old people,' she said. I laughed it off, and made my 'we are young' joke. Louise sat with us for a while, then along came one of the carers, named

Zoe (a different Zoe to the one who had come to the flat). Louise said to Bonnie, 'We are showing *The Sound of Music* in the other room. Would you like to go and see it?' 'Yes,' said Bon eagerly. 'Well, Zoe will take you.' Bonnie stood, put her arm through Zoe's, and let Zoe lead her off. She walked slightly stooped and bent to the side, though not too much. In that moment, I realised how much she had deteriorated physically. I watched her go, and she didn't look back.

Louise said to me quietly, 'This is where you evaporate out.' We went down to the office to do essential paperwork – consent forms to sign. Louise hugged me hard, and I felt the tears come. She told me again that I would suffer more than Bonnie, that I would have good days and bad days. I said I was so pleased with the way Bonnie seemed to have settled down.

'Yes,' said Louise, 'but she knows something is going on, that she is somewhere different. You mustn't let that worry you. It's always like that. When a resident settles well, it usually takes two to four weeks. If they have not settled after a month, we become worried. But from everything I have seen of Bonnie today, she is behaving exactly as we would expect.'

I felt reassured. I said I still had nagging doubts that I had put Bonnie into Sundial too soon. Louise said, 'You have done absolutely the right thing. Some people wait and wait and act when there's a crisis, and then it's really difficult.'

I left. I knew there was one major hurdle of the day left: walking into the empty flat. (I'd told Monika to take the evening off.) When I got to Marylebone station, it was pouring with rain. Sensible people were sheltering. I walked out into the rain. It matched my mood perfectly.

The tears began to prick at the back of my eyes even before I put the key into the lock. Once inside, I let them come. I cried easily. Moments of calm, then more tears. After half an hour or so, I felt them well up more strongly than ever. I hurried into the bathroom, buried my face in a towel and howled and howled. I had never done that before in my life. Only after the howling did I begin to feel a little better.

I will howl again, many times over, in the weeks and months to come. This has been the worst day of my life. I was prepared for it, which did not make it any easier. From this moment I am alone, without my Bonnie. We have both started a new life, without each other. John and Bonnie as a couple no longer exist, something I would have sworn would never be possible.

Chapter 15

Louise phoned late yesterday afternoon to say Bonnie had settled in fine, had already made friends, and had just had dinner with a male admirer! It made me so happy to hear that. Was I jealous? Not one bit. If Bonnie is happy, then I am happy.

I thought I would wake up vastly relieved this morning. But it was awful. The empty bed alongside me. I looked across to where I had seen her sleeping face yesterday. Just emptiness now. Her absence was tangible. I felt as if I could reach out and touch her even though I couldn't see her.

My overwhelming feeling on this Day One is of emotion at how trusting she was yesterday. She didn't ask me a single question. Where are you taking me? What is this place? Why are we in a single room? Not one single question. She trusted me totally. If I was taking her away somewhere, then it was the right thing to do.

Monika said a sensible thing this morning. 'John, she's very ill.' I keep forgetting that. I keep thinking of her as normal, and beating myself up for doing what I have done to her. But she has dementia. Brother David just rang. 'You have done the best possible thing you could do for the woman you love,' he said. Julie rang from Sundial to say Bonnie is fine. How can things be going this well? 'Remember,' said Julie, 'people with dementia live only in the moment, the now.' That would explain why she is content. But will it stay that way? Louise advised me not to visit today – give it a day – then go on Thursday. That is what I will do. Go out tomorrow. Will she recognise me? Will she remember who I am? Will she challenge me about why she is there?

Lunchtime. Louise has just called and we had a long, long chat. She was due to ring this evening, but she knew I would be anxious about how things were going. There have been a few small ups and downs, she said. Everything was going fine last night until bedtime. The care staff had real difficulty persuading Bonnie to get undressed and ready for bed, and it had been similar this morning. Bon had got angry: 'Everybody has been telling me what to do. I can do this.' Louise wanted to know if this was how Bonnie behaved at home, and the same sort of things she said. I said it absolutely was, 100 per cent. She said she was pleased, because that meant Bon was not reacting badly to being at Sundial – it was just a continuation of her behaviour at home.

Louise said she and her team would work on this and try to resolve it. Then she said something totally revelatory. 'When I met Bonnie for the first time last week, I was fairly sure she was ready to come to Sundial. Now, after witnessing her behaviour last night, I am totally sure. There is no question you have made the right decision. This problem with dressing and undressing is a tipping point. It is not something that you could be expected to handle.' I said I had been handling it, with varying degrees of failure, probably for the last couple of years.

'That's impossible, John. You couldn't go on like that, either for your sake or Bonnie's. You obviously wanted to keep her at home for as long as you could, but actually you could have brought her to us earlier than you did, six months even. Believe me, she needs professional care.'

Such a relief to hear that.

*   *   *   *

Almost 48 hours on, the emotion I cannot get out of mind is how trusting she was, how she just let me lead her out of the flat, unquestioning, wheeling a suitcase, onto a train, and out to Sundial. Not a single question. I knew I wasn't bringing her back. I knew she was leaving our flat ('the Suchet love nest', one of my cameramen once called it, much to our amusement) for the last time.

How can that have happened? It was never part of the plan, never the way it was supposed to happen.

I go out to Sundial today, this afternoon. It'll be the first time I have seen her there. How will she react? Will she recognise me? Will she ask me where I have been? Louise's advice is to play it absolutely normally, as if I am just coming back to the flat after a day at work. No surprises, chocolates, flowers. Parachute in.

Be prepared, Louise warned. She might well complain about the place, about all the old people around. Brush it off, and tell her you've just got back from one of your Beethoven research trips. That'll give her something to focus on and react to. Even that advice is pretty sad.

I was absolutely dreading it. I walked in with my heart in my mouth. I went up to the second floor, keyed in the number code, and entered the wide corridor of Reminiscence. I looked through the window of Louise's office. Her face broke into a broad smile when she saw me, she waved, and then her waving arm began to point over my head. I turned round and there was Bonnie, standing right behind me.

I turned, her face lit up, and she said, 'There you are! I've been waiting for you!' My determination to make it low-key went out of the window. I threw open my arms and we had a lovely hug.

Can you believe that? Arm in arm, we walked down to her room. I told her how pleased I was to be back, she said she was pleased too. In her room, I said how much I liked it, and she agreed. 'How about a walk round the grounds?' I suggested. 'Yes,' she said. With no resistance she let me put her fur hat on her head and her favourite 'puffy' coat. We walked, took in some fresh air, then back inside, where a pianist was leading a sing-song. Carers danced with residents. Bon and I sat in easy chairs. She beat time happily to the music.

Still no questions, no doubts. She appeared content. *Bless 'em all, Bless 'em all, Bless 'em all / The Long and the Short and the Tall ...* The pianist played as the residents sang along. A very elderly lady with what seemed like a permanent scowl walked past Bon and me, her face lifted into the smallest hint of a smile, and she said, 'I know other words to that – *Sod 'em all, Sod 'em all, Sod 'em all ...*' and she walked away with a mischievous grin on her face.

Carol, events organiser, saw us and said, 'Come and help me sort out all these flowers.' We went downstairs with her, and there was a table groaning with bouquets of flowers donated by Sainsbury's – bouquets they hadn't managed to sell. An elderly male resident was walking round a group of women, handing out single yellow roses. Carol picked out individual flowers and handed them to Bonnie to put into a vase. In a quiet moment I mentioned to Carol that I thought flowers were banned in Reminiscence. 'Absolutely,' she said. 'These are for Assisted Living.' She leaned forward. 'First floor, where they know flowers are for looking at, not eating.' And she chuckled. That's one thing I wasn't expecting in this place. Humour.

Still Bonnie appeared to be content, and I couldn't wipe the stupid grin from my face. Upstairs again, a little wander together, then a carer came to distract Bonnie while I 'evaporated out'. I watched her go, as I had on Tuesday, but this time there were no tears.

I sat with Louise for half an hour. I could not curb my relief and pleasure. She concurred, but warned me that things could change – even in a few weeks' time. I understood, secretly praying they wouldn't.

This morning, Friday, Alison my Admiral Nurse has come to see me. I told her how well things had gone, how I had hardly dared hope for such a result. She was pleased for me, but like Louise she warned me against thinking things had settled forever. But her emphasis was on me, rather than Bonnie. I asked her if the grief I felt would ever go. 'No,' she said, 'and it's important you don't try to run away from it.' Then she said something very wise. 'Grief is always there. It's like a wound. In time it heals, but it leaves a scar for life.'

Of course that's right. I have lost my Bonnie, now physically as well as mentally. She is still there, in Sundial, and that is the unique nature of this dreadful disease, dementia. But I am in mourning for her as surely as if she had died. That grief will stay with me until the end of my life.

* * * *

3.30 pm Friday. I have just received this text from Louise: *Right at this moment your wife is dancing the hokey-cokey with residents in Assisted Living and Reminiscence. Carol has taken photos, so will send over later!!!! Louise*

How can this be happening? Funnily enough I was just beginning to feel the slow burn of loneliness this afternoon. Lots to do, e-mails to send, after the busy last few days. Now nothing. I started pacing the flat. Then Louise's text arrived.

I will go to the park with the skipping rope and exercise myself stupid.

Later I watch television alone. *Strictly Come Dancing*. We watched the last series together. I glance across at Bonnie's chair, empty. It's fine, till they start singing some soppy music. Suddenly, without warning, the tears come.

I was in my charity's office discussing the upcoming conferences, and Diana Melly was there, manning the phone. Her late husband, the famous George, had dementia. She asked me how I was, and I said that there was no telling when the tears would come.

'You get ambushed by grief,' she said. A friend of hers had come up with the expression. 'Grief ambushes you.' What a perfect description that is. It really does ambush you. Just when I thought everything was fine this evening, it ambushed me.

* * * *

It's a week on, and Bonnie is part of the Sundial community. Hard to believe it, but she has settled right in. I went out this morning, and there she was, sitting on a sofa having a doze. I sat down gently next to her. She woke up, saw me, and a huge smile spread across her face. Still no questions. I said how good it was to be back, and she said yes.

She now knows the other residents. There is one old lady who is a grouchy miserable old thing (the one who sang *sod 'em all, sod 'em all*). When the carer tried to get her to take her pills for her diabetes, she was having none of it. 'Sod off. Bugger off.' Bon looked at me and cast her eyes to heaven. 'Take no notice,' she said.

I am getting to know the residents too. There are several who are Bonnie's age or younger. Pat, a former actress, has dementia that brings on epileptic fits. I'm not sure how old she is, but she's younger than Bon. Roger has dementia and advanced Parkinson's, and he is 57. James has Pick's disease, which affects the frontal and temporal lobes. He is 65, and used to be a television writer and director; now he cannot form a coherent sentence. Reminiscence is not just for the elderly; it is for people with dementia, and dementia is no respecter of age.

A woman came to give an exercise class to the residents. She arranged chairs in a circle, as carers brought residents to sit. It was simple basic movements, without getting out of the chair. Bonnie, once world champion 'keep fit and exercise every day' fanatic, dozed off. It brought tears to my eyes.

I had a chat with Louise in her office before leaving. 'She has already become one of us, and we adore her,' she said. I marvelled again at the lack of questions. 'I don't think she will now,' said Louise. 'She has settled. We still have problems with dressing and undressing, and she is not sleeping very well. But she is relaxed and happy.'

Should I really be that surprised? Isn't that just how my Bonnie is? Always utterly trusting and cooperative.

She has developed swollen ankles and feet. Nothing serious, said Louise. She got the doctor to look at it, and Bon is on antibiotics. If she had been at home, I would have had to book an appointment with our GP, probably for several days hence, maybe even next week, then get the prescription filled. Bon has already been seen by a doctor and is on Day Two of the antibiotics.

If ever I needed proof she was in the right place, that was it. Everything Louise said, about fitting in, being relaxed, confirmed it. Back to the empty flat. But remember, John, where you were a week ago. Utterly dreading what the next hours would bring. Now you can smile. Come on, smile. Damn you, smile.

✳ ✳ ✳ ✳

I went for a walk in Regent's Park this morning, the first such walk without Bonnie. I knew I shouldn't, but I allowed my feet to lead me to the spot deep in the park where, years ago, we decided our ashes would fertilise the soil together one day. Absurd romantic notion, I know. But that's what we did. (I was the ringleader, it's true.)

I stood there and had a cry. Got back to the flat to find Monika clearing out Bon's dressing table. Had to be done. Around 40 lipsticks and 20 jars of cream, Monika said, now in a rubbish bag. My heart sank. Years ago, Bon announced one Sunday she would tidy up her dressing table drawers. I teased her and she took it in good grace, even letting me photograph the rare event. More tears.

This is mourning, isn't it? Grieving for someone who has died? Yet I will go out to Sundial and see Bon in a couple of days and give her a big hug. I cannot get my mind round it.

This afternoon I do the first of four dementia speeches (with my charity, I whittled the number down to four). I am dreading it. I will not be able to stop the tears, and that is not manly. I don't mind crying in private, but in public it is wimpish.

I have an idea. Instead of doing the speech, why don't I get on a plane to Tahiti?

* * * *

Carol from Sundial called this morning. Last night Bonnie watched a musical on the telly, then joined in a Hollywood sing-song. She has integrated, made friends, said Carol. Still no questions, where's John, what is this place?

I found myself half-apologising to Carol for not having been out to Sundial for a couple of days. 'You mustn't feel like that,' she said. 'Some people come every day. It defeats the object. You need to let the person integrate. Also, don't forget, it is respite for you. You need the break.'

There it is, spelled out and finally filtering through my thick skull. I *am* rather enjoying the freedom – freedom to do what I like, when I like, and freedom from worrying about Bonnie. Just been for a short walk in the park. Slightly easier than yesterday. Maybe tomorrow it'll be slightly easier still.

I am tired, though, which has surprised me. Very tired. Exhausted, almost. You'd think I'd be racing around now, doing all the things I haven't been able to do, catching up on all the things I've been wanting to do.

But I'm not doing that. What I feel like doing is getting into bed, having a good cry, and sleeping for a hundred years. (Or flying to Tahiti.)

* * * *

I howled in Tardan, of course, like a wounded bear. It was a wonderful Gascon three-day wedding. Bonnie and I had been to Philippe and Cathy's wedding more than a decade ago, now here I was at our neighbour's daughter's wedding, without her. I was swept up from the moment I arrived, of course, and my hand was never left without a glass in it. I showed everyone a photo I'd taken of Bonnie in Sundial with a contented smile on her face.

There was laughter, music, dancing, eating, drinking. The wedding dinner began at six in the evening and ended at four the next morning. The lunch on day three, in the neighbour's barn right next door to Tardan, began at noon and ended (for me, at least) at 10pm. There are two widows in our village. They took it upon themselves to make sure I always had company. I was not about to complain.

But there was still the silent empty house to come back to each night. Bonnie's clothes hanging in the bedroom, that dining table with no one sitting at it and no sound of laughter, too many memories, just too many memories. All the time I was aware that the way I was behaving in the house and what I was thinking was exactly as it would be if Bonnie had died. Yet I knew I would be seeing her the day I got back.

On my return I got to Sundial quite late, around six o'clock. The residents were having their evening meal. Louise took me to Bon. I saw her sitting at a table with a couple of other residents, stooped, sipping soup, looking so different to the vibrant Bonnie I knew and loved. I had been away for three full days, hadn't seen her since the previous week. How would she react? Anger? Disappointment? Sadness? Or just blank?

I went towards her. Louise tapped her on the shoulder and said, 'Look'. She turned, saw me, let out a yelp, and laughed out loud. She stood. 'Ah, what a wonderful surprise! Oh, it's wonderful, wonderful! Look, I'm crying I'm so happy!' And she was. That made two of us.

Louise set two places at a nearby table and we ate alone. She kept smiling at me, but asked nothing, absolutely nothing. Through the window, she could see a steady stream of cars. That was all she commented on. But I could tell she was relaxed because she was with me. I kept telling her how well she looked and how good her appetite was.

Afterwards we sat on a soft sofa and watched a DVD of *My Fair Lady*. She kept drifting off to sleep. Finally I told her I was just going to spend a penny, alerted one of the carers, who distracted her while I went to sit with Louise in her office.

'She is fine, absolutely fine,' Louise said. There had been a couple of incidents – Bon had got angry with one of the women residents, clutching her on the arms. 'But that is normal,' Louise said, 'there are bound to be difficult moments. But all in all, she has settled in very well indeed. She hasn't mentioned your flat, or house in France, or what this place is, or anything. Believe me, it could have been a lot more difficult.'

I got back to the flat quite late. Empty, of course, but I am sort of used to it now. I am adapting, little by little, to life without my Bonnie.

✻ ✻ ✻ ✻

It is two weeks and a day since Bonnie went in to Sundial. I have just spoken to Louise. Bonnie has had her best day yet. She seems to be forming a relationship with Zoe, one of the lead carers. Zoe did personal hygiene with Bonnie this morning, shower and dressing, and it went better than ever before.

But here is the truly remarkable thing. Louise told me a new resident moved in this morning, and Bonnie has been asking her if she is all right. She has begun, in a small way, to care for her. *That* is my Bonnie! She's a natural carer, a born nurturer.

✻ ✻ ✻ ✻

A natural carer. Most certainly. When Bonnie's younger brother Bill was a toddler (she's three years older than him), she and he had a childish disagreement. He decided to climb on to the bedroom windowsill, but slipped. His sister dashed to the rescue, just managing to grab an ankle and prevent him from falling into the bushes below. She called for their mother, and called again, and again. Finally, realising she was in charge of the situation, she thought about it for a moment, then let him go. He suffered nothing more than a few scratches and hurt pride, and the whole family – Bill included – roared with laughter when Bon told the story at Bill's 60th birthday party in the US a few years ago.

* * * *

You don't often laugh out loud at anything to do with Alzheimer's disease, but I certainly did this morning. I read on the *Daily Mail* website that there's a report out today criticising lack of support for patients with Alzheimer's, compared to that available for those with cancer. Yeah, yeah, we know that, and that something has got to be done about it. But what made me laugh out loud was a comment from a reader who lives in Brazil.

He said a doctor there had said that investment in male virility medication and implants for women was five times more than was being invested in curing Alzheimer's. In the future, said the doctor, we will have old ladies with big breasts and old men with permanent erections, but they will not remember what their purpose is.

Got to laugh, haven't you?

I was still chuckling when I got on the train out to Sundial, and then for the first time realised I was not entirely dreading the visit. I expected Bonnie to greet me as she had last time, with evident pleasure, and again not to ask any questions. She had settled, and I did not expect there to be any change.

That didn't stop a small flutter in the stomach as I programmed in the code to let me onto the second floor. I saw her immediately, in her favourite white cashmere cardigan (the one I managed to shrink), walking along the wide corridor. I moved towards her, she saw me, looked bewildered for a moment, then cried out with joy, extended her arms, and said, 'I am so happy, so happy to see you! Look, you have made me cry!' And there they were, real tears coursing down her cheeks.

The visit went perfectly. I walked round the garden with her, petting Benny the retriever who belonged to the Sundial director, and enjoying the warm sun of late summer. Then into the bistro on the ground floor for a hot chocolate and cappuccino (yes, *déjà vu*). All the time she was calm and relaxed. There are a couple of parakeets (or some such) in a gilded cage. We watched them, laughing at their busy-ness and constant cackle. I told her to watch me as I walked towards the cage to see if I could stroke one. It stepped back, opened its beak and charged at my finger. I got it away from the psychotic bird in the nick of time. Bon loved it.

At one point I broke my own rule, told her I had forgotten my name, and asked her if she could remember it. 'You're stupid,' she said, laughing out loud, but said nothing. I asked her again. 'Of course I remember your name,' she said, 'John Something.' We both laughed.

Back up on the Reminiscence floor, Zoe told me that Bonnie walks around the corridors and large reception rooms all day, but is perfectly content. Even at meals, she said, Bon would finish her food and instantly get up and begin to wander. Just like in the flat, I said. But again Zoe stressed she was not distressed. We both agreed that on the whole she had settled in pretty much as well as it is possible to do in a strange new place with elderly disoriented people.

I left content. When I reached Baker Street, I went into the café where we would stop every morning for hot chocolate after the walk in Regent's Park. Another first. I was initially a little sad, but soon got over it.

Back in the flat, I decided I should do a little laundry. I got my towels and clothes out of the bin and sorted them according to colour. Domestic god, eh? That'll shock Monika.

✳ ✳ ✳ ✳

Brother David rang and said, Come and have dinner, just you and me, we'll pop out locally. He lives in Docklands, near Tower Bridge. Over a glass of wine, he said, 'Leave the flat, leave Chiltern Court. There are too many memories. We were kids there, for goodness sake! You mustn't cling to the past, you must move forward.' If that rather took me aback, what he said next hit me like a sledgehammer. 'Bonnie has a new life. She is in a new place, with new people. She may not have chosen it, but that is what has happened. You need a new life too.'

The thought of leaving Chiltern Court had simply never occurred to me, not once in all the years I had been living there. Nor had the rationalisation that Bonnie had a new life. I hadn't thought about it in that way. David went on, 'Why not move down here? It would be lovely to have you as a neighbour. Imagine, pick up the phone, fancy a coffee, fancy a beer?'

He registered the shock on my face. Pouring more wine, he said, 'No rush. Don't rule it out, that's all.'

* * * *

Angels exist. Halloween night at Sundial, and the carers had organised a party. They invited me and I said I would go, though frankly I wasn't really looking forward to it. A party at an old people's home. It sounded pretty grim. You can almost imagine the scenes of enforced jollity.

In the event, it was one of the most remarkable nights of my life. Exaggeration? No, I don't think so. All the carers were dressed as witches, naturally, but they were *really* good witches. The costumes were amazing. Also they distributed witches' hats, clip-on horns, evil masks, to residents. It meant everybody – carers, residents, everybody – had a permanent smile on their faces.

The professional entertainer was a one-man disco, playing hits from the last 20 years and singing to them. Sounds grim, again, but actually he was rather good.

And so the dancing began. The elderly and infirm from Assisted Living (first floor) and those with dementia from Reminiscence (second floor), gathered in the ground-floor hall. It could have been so grotesque. If Hollywood tried to recreate it, that is what it would have been. Exaggerated, bizarre, several flying over the cuckoo's nest. But it was not.

The carers – magnificent witches – worked their way round the room, pulling residents onto the dance floor. Initial reluctance gave way to smiles, as more and more of them took to the dance floor. It was those smiles. You have to have been there to see how faces lit up, years dropped away.

One 85-year-old started kicking her legs out, then revealed to everybody she had once been a professional dancer. Another seized the microphone and said she had once been a singer.

There were two men in wheelchairs, neither able to stand alone. On several occasions two carers went to them, lifted them gently to their feet, danced with them, holding them steady, then eased them back into their chairs. The men's faces were ecstatic. They were standing! They were moving their hips to the music! I watched with tears running down my cheeks.

Still the carers danced, with resident after resident. In between they checked everyone had a drink in their hands. I sat with Bonnie, and we danced. She looked embarrassed, but put her arms round me and let me lead her. She laughed constantly. I couldn't help thinking of the first time we had ever danced together. It was back in the 1970s, when I coveted her and she had pretty much no idea who I was. It was at a party in our house. I asked her to dance. I could barely move for the pounding of my heart. We didn't touch. She looked me in the eye, and very slowly swayed her hips to the music, her arms slightly away from her body and her hands turned out. I can see it as clearly now as I could more than 30 years ago. I thought then – and still do – that it was one of the most erotic things I had ever seen.

Now she was looking at me, still smiling, not quite sure how to move. So I held her tight, and just let our bodies move together.

Next to us, in an easy chair, was a very old man with a shock of white hair. He watched the witches dancing and there was a look of lost youth on his face, a longing. But the smile never stopped. I wondered what he was remembering. Wartime dance conquests? Probably. Each time a witch came to him to ask if he was all right and if he needed anything, he took her by the hands, pulled her towards him, and puckered his lips. Each time, the witch leaned forward, puckered her lips, then just very slightly turned her face so he kissed her cheek. I swear he began the evening looking about 95, and ended it looking 45.

Those witches, those carers, those women, are angels angels angels. Full stop.

Chapter 16

I went down to Tardan in November 2009, again *tout seul*. But this was different to the wedding, when I stayed for only three days and every day was taken up with fun and laughter. This was to be for 10 days, my first substantial stay without Bonnie, and I was dreading it. I had a chat with Louise out at Sundial a couple of days before, and told her how much I was dreading it. 'Then why are you going?' she asked. That took me by surprise. It had never occurred to me not to go. For the past 20 years, whenever we had some time available, Bon and I would go to Tardan.

On the train back home, I thought about what she had said. In my heart of hearts, I knew what the truthful answer was. To check the roof wasn't leaking, to check no family of mice had decided to take up residence, to make sure there were no pipes leaking, to water the flowerbeds if they looked dry. There was another reason, of course. I wanted to know how I would get on without Bonnie. Would I derive any comfort from all the memories in that house we loved so much? I suppose I knew the answer before I even got there. The question was how bad would it be.

The answer: very bad indeed. I had no idea how bad. Take the net curtain that covered the kitchen door glass, for example. What could be more boring than a frigging net curtain, for God's sake? Not this one, though. I remember how we measured the door, then bought the curtain at John Lewis in London. Bonnie set up her grandmother's old Singer sewing machine and shortened it by just the right amount. We took it down to Tardan, slipped it through the rod I had screwed to the top of the door (getting the holes right first time), and it was perfect.

'I know, let's wash it,' Bonnie said, 'freshen it up.' She put it in the washing machine, ironed it, we hung it up … and it had shrunk by three or four inches. We were gutted. 'I should have hand-washed it,' she said. 'Doesn't matter,' I replied. 'It's a bit short, but so what?' She shook her head. 'I know, I'll wash it again, by hand this time, I won't iron it, we'll hang it up wet and stretch it.' 'Yeah, by which time it'll be the size of a handkerchief,' I said helpfully.

She washed it again, hung it up wet, we stretched it, it dried, and it was perfect. It has hung there, perfect, for 15 years or so. I have not thought about it since the day we did all that. But I looked at it on the first day of my solitary visit to Tardan and the tears instantly came. Ambush.

That dining table. Ambush. Dad's consulting room chandelier, a grim dark oak light fitting which my brothers and I all remember from our childhood, and all agreed to give to charity after Dad died. 'Tardan,' said Bon, 'it'd be perfect in Tardan.' 'Where would it hang?' I asked. 'There's nowhere, not a single ceiling that's high enough.' 'Above the staircase,' she said, 'over the stairwell.' 'There's no electricity there,' I said, closing the discussion. 'Then get an electrician to put it in,' she said, and that chandelier found its home. I looked up at it. Ambush.

I opened a cupboard door and reached in for an anorak. On the shelf, I saw her Mum's straw hat Bonnie was wearing when we she stood outside Baltimore Washington airport, waiting for me almost 30 years ago, the paper flowers faded now by the strong French sun.

I walked from room to room, surrendering to grief and self-pity. I howled, the raucous sound reverberating off ancient walls that had heard nothing but laughter for 20 years. I went out on to the terrace and I could *hear* the voices and laughter, *see* Bonnie lying on the lounger. Ten days of this, I thought. Great.

The following day, I decided to call Sundial to see how Bonnie was. A carer picked up the phone, told me Bonnie was fine. 'In fact, she has just walked past the office. Would you like to speak to her?' I heard her call out to Bonnie, tell her John was on the phone, and lead her into the office. 'Here, Bonnie, take this, it's John. I'll be back in a minute.' I heard Bonnie's little gasps as she struggled to understand what to do with the phone. I called out her name, hoping she would hear my voice coming out of the earpiece. But those little gasps kept coming as she turned the receiver over in her hand. 'Darling, darling, it's me, John, it's me.' I was getting desperate. I could hear her anguish. With utter relief I heard the carer return. 'Oh dear, I'm sorry, Bonnie, here you are darling, hold this to your ear.'

I spoke and the little gasps turned to joy. 'Oh John, hello, hello, it's good to hear your voice. I …' She struggled to put a sentence together but the words wouldn't come. I kept talking, trying to keep my voice as normal as possible, though my throat had shrunk to about a tenth of its size.

I was standing in the small study, next to the kitchen. For more than a decade, before the second renovation, it had been our bedroom. I looked to where our bed had stood, and imagined all that had happened there, the moments of joy, intimacy, togetherness. How could I reconcile that with the small broken voice on the other end of the phone? The carer finally took the receiver away from her, I heard a few mumbled words, then the line went dead. I physically sank to my knees.

This cannot go on, I decided. I tried to project into the future. In a year from now, or two, or three, would things change and would I actually derive comfort from being down here? The answer, I was convinced, was no. What if I proceeded with the original intention of passing the house to the boys, so they could bring their children down here, then I would come as a guest? Would I derive comfort from that? Again I was convinced the answer was no. All of us on the terrace, surrounded by shrubs and trees planted by Bon, and Bon wasn't there? Would I derive comfort from that? Not in a million years.

Monday morning came, Day Four of my visit, and my sadness had become despair. The weather didn't help. It was pouring, great rods of rain bouncing off the terrace. I stood there gazing across the grass. 'Don't worry, it's good for the garden,' Bonnie used to say, 'and you won't have to water.' I had never felt such total, utter despair, as if there was nothing, *nothing*, that could redeem it.

It's difficult to put into words what happened next, but I felt something build up in my head until I thought it would burst. Not words, but an overwhelming urge, as if I was being given an instruction. Sounds bizarre, and I am struggling to find an apt description, but it was as if my decisions, my actions, were being taken out of my hands. Maybe it is what religious converts feel at the moment of conversion. I wouldn't know. But something was happening in my head, something that made me completely certain of what to do next.

I threw an anorak over my shoulders, and walked next door to talk to the neighbours, Raymonde and Michou. They were sitting round the table with their daughter and her new husband – the young couple whose wedding I had come to two months previously. We made a little small talk, and then I said I had made a decision. I had decided to sell up. I knew I needed to close the door on an era of my life. There were stunned faces around me.

That evening, I broke the news to Jean-Pierre and Claudette. Their jaws dropped. Jean-Pierre's eyes moistened, and I saw Claudette set her jaw to avoid showing emotion. She mentioned a few hard practicalities, which actually I was quite grateful for, then suddenly her face softened in a way I had never seen before. 'Let me have something, something from the house that I can always look at and think, That belonged to John and Bonnie.'

The three of us walked round the house together. I gave Claudette a hand-painted fruit bowl that Bonnie loved. It always stood in pride of place and in full view. What was the alternative? I should take it to London and feel sad every time I looked at it? We went upstairs. No reason, just to do a sort of tour of the house Jean-Pierre had been born in (on the same day as me, one year earlier), and of which for 20 years

Bonnie and I had had custody. In our magnificent bedroom, once the dirty dusty attic, a flash of white caught my eye. It was the statuette of the Virgin Mary we'd found on our first viewing of the house. I picked it up and handed it back to Jean-Pierre.

Momentous day. It was only later I realised it was 30th November, four years to the day since Atlanta.

✳ ✳ ✳ ✳

Back in London, I had a session with my Admiral Nurse Alison. I told her how sad I had been in the house. I said something rather irrational, that I felt a sort of resentment towards the house that after all I had done for it over the years, it had finally made me so sad. 'The house was helping you grieve,' she said wisely.

I am so pleased she said that. It meant that although the Tardan era was over, all the good memories could remain intact, without being replaced by bad ones. The house, Alison was saying, had in a sense come to my rescue. It had helped me grieve, then led me to do the right thing.

It was a turning point. I had made a decision to close the door – literally, I suppose – on the past and move forward. You can guess what that led to. I phoned brother David when I got home.

✳ ✳ ✳ ✳

Louise e-mailed me to say one of the carers had noticed that Bonnie was pulling at her necklace and, rather than risk breaking it, she had managed to remove it while getting Bon ready for bed. 'Don't worry, it's in our safe. I just didn't want you to wonder where it had vanished to. I'll give it to you next time you come out.'

And so I brought the little gold and diamond necklace home and returned it to its box for the first time since Venice.

✳ ✳ ✳ ✳

I have found a new flat. It is in Docklands, about 15 minutes' walk from my brother David. It is on the river and has spectacular views. It is larger than our flat in Chiltern Court, but has just one enormous reception room. A complete change of lifestyle. I have to brace myself now for the day I walk out of here for the last time. It may be easier than I fear. Bonnie has already done it. This flat was John and Bonnie, just as Tardan was. Time for someone else to enjoy Tardan, time for someone else to enjoy our flat.

'Bonnie's clothes need sorting out, a lot will have to go,' Monika said to me. I had known deep down that would have to be done one day, but had managed to put off thinking about it. I told her to just do it, as she had the dressing table. Don't even tell me, I said, just do it.

One day last week, she did six runs to the charity shop. Yesterday, walking to the station to go out and see Bon, I passed the charity shop and saw Bon's things in the window. Ambush. Mother and father of all ambushes. When I go to the station now, I walk on the other side of the street.

My penfriend Jim has e-mailed me from Bolton. I have to go to Manchester next week to record some *Countdown* programmes, and I have invited him to be in the studio audience. His e-mail apologises for sounding vein *[sic]*, asks if he can bring his friend Ann Gina, says he'll drive into the city on one of the main arteries.

I had to read it twice, and then collapsed in laughter. But it wasn't really all that funny. He has been diagnosed with a leaking heart valve and needs major surgery. (He just likes puns.) He is on beta-blockers and has been told to dial 999 the moment he feels any dizziness, chest pain or breathlessness. I told him he didn't need beta-blockers, he just needed to stop thinking of Angelina.

On a very slightly more serious note, as I had been warned, being a carer can kill.

✳ ✳ ✳ ✳

Bonnie greeted me today in the usual happy way. Then she said, 'I wish I could see you more often, that would make me so happy.' You can imagine what that did to me. Broke me up inside. I stayed with her a couple of hours. She seemed content, though was reluctant to sit still for more than a couple of minutes. She is much happier doing her walking. Our conversation is lively, but makes no sense. I left, drained and depressed. This could go on for years.

Should I go more often? If Bon wants it, then how can I even question it? I'm just slightly worried about what it'll do to me. Sometimes the depression consumes me, and one day it could consume me totally, and that would be that. Then I'd be no use to her at all.

✳ ✳ ✳ ✳

I can remember as if it were yesterday the very first time I ever set eyes on Bonnie back in 1971. I was standing by a window in the front room of our house in Henley, a room that looked out over the end of the cul-de-sac.

I glanced through the window. A young blonde woman was pushing a baby buggy. I could say to you that my heart stopped, I held my breath, my eyes widened. But I really don't recall what happened to me. What I can say, without any hesitation or doubt whatsoever, is that it was a *coup de foudre*. Poets write about it, singers warble about it. It happened to me in that instant. The proverbial bolt of lightning struck.

I didn't know it at the time, but I had found my Bonnie, the love of my life.

She is still the love of my life, and she always will be. The last few years have been difficult and distressing. Dementia, as I have said, is a thief.

But it cannot steal my memories, and those I will carry with me for ever. If I give in, succumb, wallow in self-pity, retreat into a shell, hibernate, give up, then that vile thief will have notched up another victim.

But it is not going to get me too. I will live and laugh. And till my last breath I will count myself the luckiest man in the world that that beautiful American East Coast blonde agreed to share my life.

Epilogue

I have a new career. It's not one I chose or ever wanted. You know me –
television journalist, reporter, newscaster, superstar. Well, some of that,
anyway. Now a new career beckons. Have I embraced it with open arms?
I have not. Do I want to get on a plane to the South Pacific instead, in
other words run away from it as far and as fast as I can? I do. But no, this
new career, this heavy mantle, has been thrown around my feeble and
unwilling shoulders.

I have become the public face of dementia.

Which is how I found myself today in a lecture hall full of healthcare
professionals, discussing how to improve the environment for people
with dementia, talking about preserving dignity for these people as they
approach the end of their lives, transforming drab, out-of-date hospital
wards and care home facilities into modern, comfortable, well-lit,
congenial surroundings. A number of people spoke, outlining ambitious
projects, and again and again I heard the words … dementia … end of
life … dignity … death …

I sat in the front row, awaiting my turn to speak. How was I going to
stand on the stage and tell these people about my Bonnie? How could I
explain to them that compared to the patients they are talking about, she
is young? She was diagnosed at the age of 64. She is not approaching the
end of her life. To know that I would be speaking about her in a forum
like this was alone enough to crack me up. The tears kept welling up, as
the professionals spoke of the difficulties and challenges of caring for
people in the advanced stages of dementia.

I now speak in public time and time again. I am used to giving talks on stage about Beethoven, or television news. But this is different. I heard myself being introduced. I walked to the podium. Behind me a huge projection of the photo of Bon and me at the RTS awards ceremony with me holding that piece of engraved glass. I looked out across a sea of expectant faces, and I spoke about Bonnie. Quietly, gently, losing my way again and again, stumbling, unprofessional, I tried to tell them what it was like to care for someone who develops dementia at a relatively early age.

I told them that unlike many carers I had a voice, and that I would use that voice to campaign tirelessly for more support for carers of loved ones with dementia, to make more Admiral Nurses available on the NHS and to stop access to them being a postcode lottery.

The most I can say is that they listened. This was not a performance, I was speaking from the heart. I was speaking about the woman I loved, who was now lost to me. As I walked back to my seat I thought to myself I had better get used to this, because this is how it is going to be from now on. There is going to be a lot more of this.

2009 was the year when dementia entered the public consciousness. The government published its first ever National Dementia Strategy in February; Sir Terry Pratchett made two television documentaries about his Alzheimer's; TV presenter Fiona Phillips made a television documentary about giving up work so she could better look after her dad who had dementia, her mum having already died with it; the *Jeremy Vine Show* on BBC Radio 2 devoted a week to dementia; and yes, I went public about my Bonnie and there was a certain amount of reaction.

A certain amount of reaction? My charity, *for dementia*, was hit by a tidal wave of e-mails from people asking if there were Admiral Nurses in their country, and if so, how they could get access to one. The answer, of course, was that there weren't any even a mile away from where I lived in London, let alone Australia or China.

My charity, with just 14 full-time employees, faced a choice. It could either embrace this welter of interest, or it could quietly walk away and pretend none of it had happened.

It chose the former course. The first decision it took was that it needed to change its name. I pointed out that in speaking in public about the charity, I found it difficult to form an elegant sentence incorporating the name: 'the charity I work for, *for dementia* …' The point was taken up by the chief executive and put to the Trustees. It was agreed that a more easily spoken name should be found, and that in this Google age dementia should be the first word in the name. A new name should also reflect the national scope of the charity, with its aim to provide Admiral Nurses and dementia training nationwide. And so in March 2010 *for dementia* became Dementia UK.

Another idea, a major project, was brought forward. For a year or more, discussions had been taking place within the charity about the creation of an Admiral Nurse Academy. Its aim would be to identify suitable fully qualified nurses early in their career and offer them specialist training in dementia care. The charity had already established contact with several universities with a view to working together. The 'Academy' would be virtual, with its website forming the major point of entry.

As a direct result of the publicity that followed my going public about Bonnie, the creation of the Academy was brought forward. On 26th May 2010, at an international dementia conference in Canterbury, I announced the establishment of the Admiral Nurse Academy.

The trustees of Dementia UK made one other decision. The Admiral Nurse Academy is to be named 'In Honour of Bonnie Suchet'.

There, my darling Bonnie, that is your legacy.

Acknowledgements

The idea for this book was put to me by Carole Tonkinson, Publisher of Harper NonFiction, who said she wanted me to tell 'the love story'. Throughout the process, she has been more than an editor – she has encouraged, guided and counselled.

Gill Paul went through the completed manuscript line by line, word by word. If the book now has a coherent structure, it is thanks to her.

I am grateful to Carole and Gill beyond words. I also wish to thank HarperCollins for offering to donate a percentage of their royalties to my charity, Dementia UK.

Barbara Stephens, chief executive of Dementia UK (formerly known as *for dementia*), and Rhonda Smith, communications consultant, have had to interrupt busy lives to deal with dozens of e-mails from me asking for information for this book, and Joy Watkins of Uniting Carers has always been on hand to send me 'Say No' potion with instructions to drink whenever the requests to speak about dementia threaten to over-whelm me.

My Admiral Nurse Ian Weatherhead, who for years has gone about his life-saving business with quiet dedication, suddenly found himself in the newspapers and on the airwaves after February 2009. Sorry for doing that to you, Ian, but you keep telling me it's for a good cause.

Finally, I wanted nothing in this book to come as a surprise to our sons, and so all five of them read it in manuscript. They complained that the photos show them in a previous era, looking seriously uncool.